The Emotionally Intelligent Clinician

Harnessing the Power of Emotional Intelligence to Transform Patient Care and Enhance Professional Success

Dr Lora Banicevic

First Edition

Published by *TEIC Publishing*

www.drlorabanicevic.com

Contents

Note To Readers

Due to printing constraints, all illustrations in this book appear in black and white. Full-colour versions, along with additional downloadable tools and resources, are available at drlorabanicevic.com on the Book Resources page.

Introduction

There was a day, not too unlike any other in the bustling life of a busy dental practice, when a particularly nervous patient reminded me of why I do what I do. She walked into my Sydney practice, Corner 32 Dental, her anxiety palpable, eyes darting around as if looking for the nearest exit. It was a familiar sight; one I've encountered countless times. As I met her in the reception area, I sought a way to ease her apprehension, reassured her that we would simply start the appointment with a chat to get to know each other and ushered her down the hall to my clinic room. We sat down opposite each other, and I initiated our conversation with, "Hi, I'm Lora, it's nice to meet you. What can I do for you today?". Her words poured out in a torrent, a mixture of fear and shame stemming from past dental experiences. She was talking quickly and loudly, jumping from one story to the next so rapidly I could barely keep up. I listened intently though, navigating her rapid narrative with empathy and patience. Once she was done, I could see that she was almost physically exhausted but satisfied and content that she had been heard. The relief on her face was obvious. It is in these moments of calm reassurance, of gentle conversation that go beyond the mere technicalities of dental care, that I am reminded of the profound impact we can have on people every day — not just in dentistry, but across all realms of healthcare. What I do in my clinic every day is not just about fixing teeth; it's about understanding fears, easing pain (both physical and emotional), and building trust. This story, among many others, fuels this book's purpose: to illuminate the necessity and power of emotional intelligence in healthcare — not only as a means of delivering exceptional patient care, but as a foundation for personal growth, emotional resilience, and long-term fulfilment in your professional life.

Hi, I'm Dr Lora, a dentist with a heart as invested in cultivating emotional intelligence as it is in promoting oral health. Since my days at the University of Sydney, where my journey in dentistry began, to the founding of my practice, Corner 32 Dental and beyond, I've been on a relentless quest for knowledge. This quest isn't just about staying abreast of the latest in dental care, which I believe is critical in all health fields — it's about understanding people. My team and I have dedicated ourselves to creating a space where compassion reigns supreme, where patients, especially the anxious ones, feel seen, heard, and valued. This commitment extends beyond the walls of my practice; it's about nurturing a holistic approach to healthcare, where developing emotional intelligence is as crucial as clinical skill, if not more so. And just as it helps patients feel seen and supported, emotional intelligence helps us as clinicians stay grounded, reduce burnout, communicate more effectively, and reconnect with the purpose that brought us into healthcare in the first place. After all, our wealth of acquired skills and knowledge will remain inaccessible if we lack the critical skill of emotional intelligence to establish rapport and build trust with our patients from the outset. This is why nearly every, if not every, job advertisement I come across for a clinician includes a request for 'excellent communication skills' or something similar. Our professional success rides on our ability to build and sustain relationships with others.

If you've ever left a shift feeling emotionally drained, wondered how to navigate conflict with grace, or simply wished for deeper connection in your work — this book is for you. It's a guide — a companion on your journey as a health professional toward harnessing the power of emotional intelligence. And it's designed to help you care not only for others, but for yourself.

In a field where emotional strain and high-stakes decisions are part of daily life, mastering emotional intelligence allows you to build resilience, manage stress more effectively, and find deeper meaning in your work. Through self-awareness, emotional regulation, and empathy that not only soothes but protects, you'll be better equipped to thrive — not just survive — in your career.

Emotional intelligence is a skill, not a talent, and it can be improved and refined with practice. In these pages, we'll explore the science of EQ — but more importantly, we'll dive into its application: how you can use it to transform patient care, achieve personal fulfilment, and enhance your professional success.

Structured to be both a learning experience and an interactive guide, the chapters unfold from understanding the basics of emotional intelligence to mastering it in your personal and professional interactions. You'll find strategies for stress management, ways to bounce back from setbacks, and techniques for building stronger, more authentic connections with patients and colleagues. Each section is punctuated with exercises, real-world scenarios, and evidence-based practices, ensuring that the insights gained are not just theoretical but immediately applicable.

To my fellow health professionals who have a desire to connect more deeply with your patients, navigate workplace challenges with confidence, and find greater fulfilment in your career, this book is for you. Whether you're a nurse, a doctor, a therapist, allied health professional or a dentist like me, the principles of emotional intelligence are universal. They are the bridge between clinical expertise and truly transformative care. With a mix of scientific research and personal anecdotes from my own experiences — especially those involving nervous patients — I hope to offer you a unique perspective on the challenges and rewards of applying emotional intelligence in your own field.

As you turn these pages, see this not just as professional development, but as a journey of personal transformation — an opportunity to cultivate a more balanced, fulfilling, and connected life with your patients, your colleagues, your loved ones, and most importantly, yourself — both within your healthcare role and beyond it. This is more than a book; it's a call to action. Let it be your stepping stone toward a career and a life enriched with emotional intelligence, where patient care becomes more impactful, communication more meaningful, and fulfilment more lasting. Together, let's embark on this journey — not just to become better healthcare professionals, but to become more empathetic, understanding, and compassionate people.

With warmth and encouragement,
Lora

Chapter 1

The Neuroscience Behind Emotional Intelligence

1.1 The Amygdala: Your Brain's Alarm System

"We don't think; we feel, we act."

— Sue Johnson

In the vast expanse of the human brain, a tiny structure no larger than an almond holds the key to some of our most profound emotional experiences. This structure, known as the amygdala, serves as our brain's alarm system — constantly scanning for threats and orchestrating our emotional and physiological responses with astonishing precision.

For those of us working in healthcare, understanding the amygdala's role in emotional regulation is not just academic — it's essential. It helps us better care for our patients under pressure and gives us insight into our own reactions in the high-stress situations we regularly face.

THE ROLE OF THE AMYGDALA IN EMOTIONAL REGULATION

The amygdala, nestled deep within the brain's medial temporal lobe, has long captivated scientists and psychologists alike for its central role in processing emotions. Its primary function is to detect and respond to stimuli that elicit feelings, particularly those related to survival such as fear. When we encounter a stressful event — an emergency on the floor, a distressed patient, a complex diagnosis — our amygdala kicks in. It assesses the threat level and triggers a response designed to protect the individual from harm. This response can manifest as a surge of adrenaline, heightened alertness, or a readiness to act — reactions that are invaluable in crisis situations.

However, the amygdala's influence extends beyond immediate physical threats. It also plays a crucial role in social and emotional perception, particularly in interpreting the emotional states of others — especially through non-verbal cues like body language or facial expressions. For us, this means that the amygdala is instrumental in recognising and responding to the subtle cues of patient discomfort or distress. It is why a nurse can walk into a room and, within moments, sense that a patient is anxious without a word being spoken.

Yet, the amygdala's rapid response system, while often beneficial, can also be a double-edged sword. In the high-stress environments of healthcare settings, the constant activation of the amygdala can lead to emotional exhaustion. Healthcare professionals are regularly exposed to situations that trigger their amygdalae — whether it's dealing with life-and-death emergencies, navigating complex interactions with patients and their families, or managing their own reactions to patient outcomes. Over time, this relentless stimulation can wear down even the most resilient individuals and the most experienced clinicians, leading to burnout and compassion fatigue.

Understanding the functions of the amygdala is the first step in managing its responses. By recognising the signs of amygdala activation — such as rapid heartbeat, shallow breathing, or a sudden feeling of alertness — we can begin to regulate our emotional reactions. This self-awareness is crucial in allowing us to remain calm and focused in the face of stress, ensuring that our decisions and actions are guided by professional judgment rather than raw emotion. Learning to pause and check in with these signals therefore allows us to respond with intention rather than react impulsively. This skill takes time and experience to build but is critical to a balanced and fulfilled career in healthcare, especially if we want to lead with calm and clarity.

Moreover, strategies for regulating amygdala-triggered responses are essential tools for healthcare professionals. Practices such as deep breathing, mindfulness meditation, and cognitive reappraisal (learning to reinterpret stressful situations) can help mitigate the amygdala's alarm signals, reducing the physiological and emotional intensity of stress reactions. These techniques enable us to access our higher, more rational, thought centres to maintain a state of calm and presence, allowing for better decision making and thereby ensuring that we can provide the highest level of care to our patients. We'll explore these and other strategies in more detail throughout the book.

Beyond these personal strategies, we must also acknowledge the power of creating or choosing a supportive work environment as vital in managing the collective amygdala response of healthcare teams. Emotional regulation is not a solo sport — team culture matters. Regular debriefings after high-stress incidents, peer support programs, and training in emotional regulation techniques can help team members process difficult experiences together and develop resilience. By acknowledging the psychological toll of their work and providing tools to manage it, healthcare organisations can protect the well-being of their team members. When leaders model emotional intelligence, they create safe, supportive spaces that reduce chronic stress and enhance both job satisfaction and patient care.

Reflection: Understanding Your Own Alarm System

Take a moment to explore your own relationship with the amygdala's response:

- *When was the last time you felt your "amygdala alarm" go off in a clinical setting? What triggered it?*
- *How did you respond? Did it feel like an intentional response, or more like a reflex/automatic response?*
- *What signs does your body give you when your stress response is activated?*
- *What tools or strategies have helped you regulate your emotional state in the past?*
- *What new approaches or habits could help you respond with greater calm and clarity next time?*

The more familiar you become with your emotional triggers and stress responses, the more power you have to lead yourself — and others — with empathy, composure, and strength.

1.2 Prefrontal Cortex: The Centre for Rational Thought

> *"Most of our conscious activity is happening in our prefrontal cortex, the part of our brain responsible for focus, handling short-term memory, solving problems, and moderating impulse control. It's at the heart of what makes us human and the center for our executive control and willpower."*
>
> — Gary Keller

When emotion surges and pressure mounts, the prefrontal cortex steps in as the brain's command centre — bringing order to chaos and allowing us to think, plan, and act with intention. This region, positioned at the very front of the brain, is the epicentre of rational thought. It processes the constant influx of information from our environment and guides us to respond with clarity, not reactivity. For healthcare professionals, this ability to regulate emotion and apply logic isn't just helpful — it's foundational. It underpins our capacity to care for others under pressure, make critical decisions, and lead with confidence and composure.

The prefrontal cortex allows us to navigate the turbulence of clinical environments, where decisions often carry weighty consequences. In moments of crisis, when the amygdala sets off an alarm, it's the prefrontal cortex that tempers the reaction — filtering through the urgency and guiding us to act with clinical reasoning. Consider an emergency room doctor faced with a critically injured patient. Despite a surge of adrenaline and urgency, it's the prefrontal cortex that takes charge, helping them prioritise, sequence, and act based on training and evidence, rather than panic.

Emotional intelligence relies on this very process: noticing our emotional reaction and pausing long enough to respond with perspective. Techniques like deep breathing, grounding, or a brief mindfulness moment can help activate the prefrontal cortex by calming the stress response and promoting clearer thinking. This doesn't mean suppressing emotions — it means recognising them and engaging the brain's executive functions to respond in a way that's both human and helpful.

Take, for example, a patient who resists treatment. It's easy to feel frustrated or impatient — a natural, amygdala-driven reaction to perceived stubbornness. But if we pause and reflect — activating the prefrontal cortex — we might instead recognise fear or confusion underlying their behaviour. Reframing these moments in a more objective or compassionate light allows us to shift from reactivity to curiosity. With this insight, we can adjust our approach, offering reassurance or clear explanations that help bridge the gap and overcome barriers to care. This process — acknowledging our emotional response, understanding its source, and choosing an intentional way forward — is the hallmark of emotional intelligence in action. Ultimately, it's about learning to pause and respond, rather than reacting on autopilot.

Importantly, the benefits of prefrontal regulation extend beyond patient care. In leadership and professional decision-making — especially when ethical grey areas arise — it's this part of the brain that helps us evaluate competing priorities, consider long-term consequences, and make values-aligned decisions. Whether allocating limited resources or navigating end-of-life care conversations, this capacity for measured, moral reasoning is critical.

Strengthening the connection between the prefrontal cortex and amygdala helps us not only stay calm under pressure but make better decisions, lead more effectively, and care more deeply. Practices like mindfulness, cognitive reframing, and regular reflective practice reinforce this connection and allow us to access both emotional and intellectual intelligence, even in the most difficult moments. These techniques — and how to implement them — will be explored in later chapters.

1.3 EQ vs. IQ: Shifting the Focus in Healthcare Professional Development

---

> *"What really matters for success, character, happiness and life-long achievements is a definite set of emotional skills – your EQ — not just purely cognitive abilities that are measured by conventional IQ tests."*
>
> — Daniel Goleman

A paradigm shift is quietly unfolding in the realm of healthcare, one that moves beyond the conventional metrics of intelligence quotient (IQ) to embrace the nuanced terrain of emotional intelligence (EQ). Healthcare professionals are increasingly realising that their personal and professional success is not solely determined by technical skills or medical knowledge but also by the ability to empathise with patients, communicate effectively, and build trust. Emotional intelligence plays a crucial role in fostering these qualities, ultimately leading to better patient experiences and outcomes. This evolution in thought doesn't diminish the value of cognitive skill — it simply acknowledges that true excellence in healthcare lies not just in what we know, but in how we connect. The shift toward emotional intelligence marks a growing recognition that empathy, communication, and the deeply human experience of connection are just as essential to healing as clinical expertise.

RETHINKING PROFESSIONAL COMPETENCE

Redefining professional competence necessitates a critical examination of what we consider the hallmarks of a successful healthcare professional. Historically, the focus has been disproportionately on theoretical knowledge and technical skill — quantifiable attributes that, while undeniably important, paint an incomplete picture of healthcare proficiency. Emotional intelligence (EI) — which includes self-awareness, self-regulation, motivation, empathy, and social skills — is equally vital. These capabilities enable clinicians to navigate the complex web of human emotion, creating environments where healing becomes not just a physical process, but an emotional journey. My own mission to shift this paradigm began in the dental chair. Time and time again, I heard patients say how much they hated going to the dentist, recounting stories laced with fear, embarrassment, shame, judgement or feeling dismissed. I wanted to change that narrative — to create experiences where patients felt heard, respected, and even surprised at how positive their visits could be. But as I moved through my career and listened to the experiences of friends, family, and colleagues in other areas of healthcare, I began to see a bigger issue. The same lack of emotional awareness, connection, and empathy was present across the entire healthcare system — not just in dentistry. That realisation became the fuel for this book. Compelling patient care stories no longer hinge solely on medical interventions, but also on the quality of the human interactions that accompany them. Patients are far more likely to trust and adhere to treatment plans when they feel understood and supported by their healthcare providers. In this light, emotional intelligence becomes more than a desirable trait — it's the missing link in how we deliver holistic care that honours the whole person, not just the diagnosis.

What's more, a strong correlation exists between high emotional intelligence in healthcare providers and a reduced risk of malpractice claims. Approximately 8% of physicians face a malpractice claim annually, with many arising from adverse events linked to communication breakdowns. Notably, studies estimate that 80% of medical errors result from miscommunication among healthcare providers and between providers and patients. By enhancing communication and fostering stronger patient relationships, high EI serves as a protective factor against such claims. When patients feel seen, heard, and respected — when they like and trust you as a person — they're far more likely to allow space for human error. They're less inclined to escalate issues and more open to resolution if something goes wrong. In many cases, it's not the mistake itself but the way it's handled that determines whether a patient lodges a complaint. Emotional intelligence helps us navigate those critical moments with transparency, empathy, and humility, which can make all the difference. Additionally, healthcare professionals with elevated EI levels are less prone to burnout — a condition associated with increased medical errors and subsequent malpractice suits. Therefore, cultivating emotional intelligence is integral to personal well-being and pivotal in mitigating legal risks, further underscoring its value in redefining professional competence.

THE CASE FOR EQ IN LEADERSHIP, EDUCATION, AND WELLBEING

The influence of EQ on leadership within healthcare settings further underscores its significance. Effective leadership, particularly in environments as dynamic and challenging as healthcare, requires more than the ability to make informed decisions. It demands an empathetic understanding of the diverse needs of patients and team members, the capacity to inspire trust and confidence, and the agility to navigate the nuances of team dynamics. Leaders endowed with high levels of emotional intelligence naturally cultivate a culture of openness, innovation, and resilience. They recognise that the strength of a team lies not just in its collective clinical expertise but in its ability to communicate, collaborate, and support one another. Such leaders are adept at motivating their teams, not through authority alone but through empathy, understanding, and the shared pursuit of excellence in patient care. Further, in today's multidisciplinary healthcare teams, effective communication and collaboration are essential. Emotional intelligence enables healthcare professionals to navigate complex interpersonal dynamics, resolve conflicts, and work cohesively towards common goals, enhancing overall team performance and patient care.

The integration of EQ into the education of healthcare professionals represents a forward-thinking approach to preparing the next generation of healthcare providers. Medical and nursing curricula, traditionally steeped in the biomedical sciences, are increasingly incorporating training on emotional intelligence but it needs to be emphasised further. This integration must take form in coursework on communication, ethics, and professionalism, complemented by experiential learning opportunities that allow students to practice empathy, teamwork, and emotional regulation in clinical settings. The goal must be to produce healthcare professionals who are not only clinically competent but also emotionally intelligent — individuals capable of forging meaningful connections with patients, navigating the complexities of healthcare delivery, and contributing to a positive workplace culture.

The journey towards emotional intelligence does not culminate with the completion of formal education though; it is an ongoing process of personal and professional development. It is easy to get caught up in continuing professional development (CPD) to enhance or learn new clinical skills, especially since university does not adequately prepare us for the real-world scenarios we face in all health professions, but lifelong EQ development is integral to career advancement and personal fulfilment in healthcare as well as ensuring professional well-being. The demanding nature of healthcare professions can take a toll on the mental and emotional well-being of practitioners. Developing emotional intelligence skills such as self-awareness, self-regulation, and resilience can help us better manage stress, prevent burnout, and maintain satisfaction in our careers. Professionals who commit to cultivating their emotional intelligence find that it not only enhances their interactions with patients but also bolsters their resilience in the face of professional challenges. Continuous learning in EQ can take many forms, from formal continuing education courses to informal learning communities among colleagues. It involves reflective practice, seeking feedback, and embracing opportunities for growth. As we advance in our careers, the cultivation of emotional intelligence remains a dynamic, evolving process, one that adapts to the changing landscapes of healthcare and the diverse needs of the populations we serve.

In essence, the shift from a singular focus on IQ to a balanced emphasis on EQ would mark a significant evolution in the field of healthcare. This necessary shift acknowledges that the art of healing is as much about understanding and connecting with the human spirit as it is about diagnosing and treating disease. It recognises that the highest standards of healthcare are achieved not solely through technical excellence but through the integration of emotional intelligence into every patient interaction, every team collaboration, and every leadership decision. As healthcare continues to navigate the complexities of the 21st century, the cultivation of emotional intelligence among healthcare professionals must guide the way towards a more compassionate, empathetic, and effective healthcare system.

1.4 Neuroplasticity and Growing Your EQ

> *"In nature nothing is hardwired, everything is livewired, everything is evolvable."*
>
> — Abhijit Naskar

"Our brains renew themselves throughout life to an extent previously thought not possible."

— Michael S. Gazzaniga

GROWING EMOTIONAL INTELLIGENCE THROUGH NEUROPLASTICITY

You've likely heard the phrase "Neurons that fire together, wire together", first used by neuropsychologist, Donald Hebb in the late 1940s. This is the basis of neuroplasticity, which in simple terms, refers to the brain's remarkable ability to adapt and change throughout our lives. Just as muscles grow stronger with exercise, our brains can rewire and form new connections in response to new experiences, learning, and environmental stimuli. This phenomenon underscores the incredible potential for growth, learning, and recovery, highlighting the dynamic nature of our brains and the capacity for lifelong development. This means that with repetition, skills that may not come naturally to us, can be learned and strengthened. This remarkable characteristic of the brain, its ability to rewire itself in response to experiences, presents a gateway to not only understanding but actively improving how we perceive, process, and respond to the emotional world around us. It is within this dynamic framework that the potential for growing one's emotional intelligence lies, offering a tangible method to augment abilities in emotional regulation and empathy through deliberate practice and learning.

At the core of this transformative process is the recognition that the brain's malleability extends to those areas pivotal for emotional intelligence, such as the prefrontal cortex and the amygdala. Targeted exercises aimed at strengthening the connections between these regions can significantly enhance an individual's capacity for emotional regulation, enabling a more adept navigation of emotional landscapes. For instance, practicing mindfulness meditation, which involves fostering an acute awareness of the present moment, encourages a more nuanced engagement with one's emotional state, facilitating a recalibration of responses to stress and emotional triggers. This practice, through repeated engagement, gradually reshapes the neural pathways, embedding a greater propensity for emotional balance and resilience.

Similarly, exercises focused on developing empathy harness neuroplasticity to deepen our understanding and connection with others. Fostering connections with others is essential for our well-being. These connections not only provide emotional support and enhance patient care but also contribute to professional growth, resilience, and overall job satisfaction. Techniques that encourage perspective-taking, for example, challenge the brain to consider and emotionally process situations from viewpoints other than our own. We are prompted to step outside our own experiences and view situations through the lens of another person. This act of cognitive and emotional stretching expands the neural circuits that underpin empathy, gradually enhancing our ability to connect with and understand the emotions of others. As these practices become embedded in our daily routines, the brain's architecture adjusts, solidifying these pathways of empathy and understanding.

PRACTICAL TECHNIQUES TO STRENGTHEN EMPATHY AND EMOTIONAL REGULATION

One effective method to do this is role-playing exercises, where we assume the perspective of a patient, colleague, or even a family member dealing with a difficult situation. By actively engaging in these scenarios, we can experience the emotional weight of a patient's fears or a coworker's frustrations, helping us to cultivate a more compassionate approach to our interactions. Another powerful technique is narrative medicine, which involves reading or listening to patient stories and reflecting on their experiences. Research has shown that storytelling activates the same brain regions used when we personally experience emotions, making it an effective tool for fostering empathy. Consider journalling about patient encounters or write from the perspective of a patient as this can also deepen your emotional connection and understanding.

Cognitive reappraisal exercises — which involve actively reframing a situation from another person's perspective — are another practical approach. For example, instead of reacting with frustration to a noncompliant patient, a clinician might pause and consider the patient's fears, socioeconomic challenges, or past medical trauma. This deliberate shift in thinking helps reduce judgment and enhances emotional connection.

Additionally, mindfulness-based techniques encourage perspective-taking by helping individuals become more aware of their own biases and assumptions. Practices such as guided meditations on compassion or exercises in deep listening train healthcare professionals to approach interactions with curiosity and openness rather than preconceptions. We will explore all these techniques in more detail in later chapters.

By consistently engaging in these techniques, the brain adapts to make empathy more instinctual. These exercises not only improve patient care but also foster stronger professional relationships, reducing workplace conflicts and enhancing overall job satisfaction. Over time, perspective-taking becomes an ingrained habit, allowing us to navigate emotionally charged situations with greater understanding, patience, and emotional intelligence.

The journey toward elevated emotional intelligence through leveraging neuroplasticity is underscored by the principle that consistent practice is key. The brain, in its adaptability, thrives on repetition and engagement. Activities such as journaling, which encourages reflective thought on emotional experiences, or participation in emotional intelligence workshops, which provide structured opportunities for emotional skill development, serve as fertile ground for this neural growth. Each encounter with these types of exercises acts as a stimulus for the brain, prompting the reinforcement and creation of new neural connections.

Moreover, the integration of emotional intelligence practices into professional development programs for healthcare professionals exemplifies the practical application of neuroplasticity in a structured learning environment. These programs, by offering a curriculum that spans the gamut from self-awareness exercises to empathy-building scenarios, cater to the comprehensive development of emotional intelligence skills. As participants engage with the material, whether through role-playing patient interactions that require empathy or navigating complex emotional scenarios that challenge their emotional regulation, the brain responds. The repeated activation of neural circuits associated with these skills leads to their strengthening, embodying the principle that through continuous learning and practice, significant increases in emotional intelligence are attainable.

In parallel, the role of feedback in this developmental process cannot be overstated. When delivered constructively and with care, feedback acts like a mirror — reflecting our emotional behaviours and responses in a way that encourages insight and growth. It becomes a critical part of the learning cycle, offering valuable perspectives we can reflect on and use to improve. When it comes to building emotional intelligence, this feedback loop helps us identify blind spots and areas for growth, shaping the focus of the tools and practices we choose to develop. Through this ongoing process of action, reflection, and adjustment — supported by the feedback of peers, mentors, and our own self-assessments — we gradually strengthen our emotional awareness and skill.

The exploration of neuroplasticity and its relationship with emotional intelligence opens a vista of possibilities for personal and professional growth. It dispels the notion that our emotional capabilities are fixed, offering instead the possibility of adaptability and change.

1.5 The Biological Basis of Empathy in Clinical Settings

> *"Empathy is the medicine the world needs."*
>
> — Judith Orloff

The neuroscience behind empathy reveals a complex interplay of neural pathways that, when activated, allow us to sense and understand the emotions of others. This capacity isn't just a desirable trait in healthcare — it's foundational. Empathy forms the backbone of meaningful patient-provider relationships and significantly influences clinical outcomes. But its impact extends far beyond the patient. When empathy is embedded in everyday practice, it enhances the emotional well-being of clinicians, strengthens team dynamics, and contributes to greater job satisfaction and professional fulfilment. In fact, clinicians who consistently practice empathy often report lower levels of burnout, stronger patient connections, and greater career success overall. Empathy, then, is not just a soft skill — it's a core component of resilient, effective, and sustainable healthcare delivery.

THE MIRROR NEURON SYSTEM: HOW EMPATHY BEGINS IN THE BRAIN

At the heart of this process is the mirror neuron system, a network of specialised neurons that fire both when we perform an action and when we observe someone else performing the same action. Discovered in the 1990s through studies on macaque monkeys, mirror neurons provide the biological basis for understanding others' emotions, intentions, and even physical sensations. When we see a patient wince in pain, for example, our mirror neurons activate as if we were experiencing that pain ourselves. This automatic, unconscious response helps us recognise distress in others and instinctively adjust our behaviour to offer comfort and support.

For healthcare professionals, the mirror neuron system is what allows us to quickly pick up on nonverbal cues — a furrowed brow, a hesitant glance, a tightening jaw — and respond with appropriate empathy. This is why an experienced clinician can walk into a room and sense almost immediately if a patient is anxious, in pain, or reluctant to speak. Our brains are wired to read these subtle signals without needing explicit verbal confirmation. This ability to intuitively "feel" what others are experiencing is crucial in healthcare settings, where patients often struggle to articulate their fears or discomfort.

But mirror neurons do more than just help us recognise emotions; they also enable us to influence the emotions of others through mirroring and emotional contagion. This is why a calm and reassuring presence can help de-escalate an anxious or distressed patient. If a patient is fearful or agitated, maintaining a composed demeanour, slowing your speech, and using open body language can subconsciously signal to their brain that they are safe, helping them regulate their emotions. This same principle applies to interactions with colleagues — staying composed in stressful situations can prevent panic from spreading and promote a culture of steady, rational decision-making.

Understanding the mirror neuron system also highlights the importance of self-awareness in emotional regulation. Just as we can absorb and reflect the emotions of others, our patients and colleagues can just as easily pick up on our stress, frustration, or impatience. This is why emotional intelligence — particularly the ability to regulate our own emotions — is essential in healthcare. If we allow ourselves to become visibly flustered or irritated, those emotions can ripple through the interaction, making patients feel more uneasy or defensive.

In the chapters ahead, we will explore practical applications of mirroring techniques — how subtle adjustments in body language, speech patterns, and emotional regulation can help diffuse tense situations and create a more therapeutic environment. Harnessing the power of the mirror neuron system isn't just about reading emotions; it's about actively shaping the emotional landscape of our interactions to foster trust, reduce anxiety, and ultimately, improve patient outcomes.

REGULATING EMOTION TO STRENGTHEN EMPATHY

True empathy extends beyond the automatic mirroring of observed emotions though. It involves a deliberate, cognitive effort to step into the shoes of another, to explore the depths of their emotional experience without losing oneself in the process. This distinction between emotional contagion, an unconscious, automatic response, and cognitive empathy, a conscious, effortful understanding, underscores the complexity of empathetic engagement in patient care. For us as healthcare professionals, the challenge lies not in merely reflecting patients' emotions but in interpreting these emotions within the context of their health experiences, thereby forging a connection that is both understanding and therapeutic.

The development of this nuanced form of empathy is contingent upon the ability to regulate one's own emotional responses, a function primarily mediated by the prefrontal cortex as discussed earlier. This regulatory mechanism ensures that we maintain a balance, allowing us to offer support to our patients without becoming overwhelmed by our own empathetic reactions. Furthermore, the capacity to differentiate between one's own emotions and those of the patient, a concept known as emotional separation, is crucial. Through practices such as reflective listening and perspective-taking exercises, we can strengthen this capacity, enhancing our ability to provide care that is compassionate, but also effective.

Often, instead of actively listening and responding to what the other person is saying, many people, and this includes healthcare providers, are simply listening for a pause in the conversation as an opportunity to interject with their own thoughts or comments, rather than genuinely engaging with the other person's message. Engaging in reflective listening, therefore, offers a powerful method for deepening empathetic engagement. This technique involves not just hearing but actively understanding and reflecting the feelings and thoughts expressed by our patients. By validating these emotions and experiences through reflective responses, we have the chance to communicate a profound sense of empathy and respect for the patient's perspective. This validation can significantly impact our patients, often serving as a catalyst for trust and openness, which are essential for effective healthcare delivery and increasing our own well-bring and satisfaction at work. In his excellent book, *The 7 Habits of Highly Effective People*, Stephen R. Covey outlines the basis of empathetic communication as *"seek first to understand, then to be understood"*. All people want is to be genuinely seen and heard before they will be able to effectively hear anything you have to say to them in return. This is why I find it is crucial when interviewing a patient for the first time, for example in a new patient examination, that the patient be allowed to express their needs, fears, concerns and wants fully before any productive conversation about their dental condition can take place. This means not only actively listening and taking note of the information the patient shares but also resisting the instinct to immediately correct, educate, or jump into problem-solving. Instead, true engagement requires establishing a solid connection first — ensuring that, at a minimum, basic trust has been formed before offering guidance or recommendations.

Perspective-taking exercises further augment the development of cognitive empathy. These exercises challenge us as healthcare professionals to consciously adopt the perspectives of our patients, to consider not just the immediate emotional reactions but the broader context of these emotions. You could ask yourself "What might this patient be feeling in this situation?" or "How would I feel if I were in the patient's shoes?" to encourage a deeper engagement with the patient's experience. Over time, regular engagement in perspective-taking exercises can help us to automatically consider and integrate patients' perspectives into our care approach, fostering a more empathetic and relationship-centred practice.

The impact of empathy on patient-provider relationships cannot be overstated. Patients who feel understood and valued are more likely to be open about their symptoms, answer questions truthfully, adhere to treatment plans, and engage actively in their care. I often joke with patients during their six-monthly check-ups about how frequently they floss — because let's be honest, most people aren't flossing nearly as much as they should. But there's an important difference between bringing lightness to a conversation and making someone feel ashamed.

Just the other day, one of my long-standing patients was in for a check-up and mentioned how much easier it had been to floss since we'd straightened her teeth. Her sister — who I hadn't seen in years because she moved away but used to be a patient of mine — had told her earlier that week, "Lora was the first dentist I ever saw who didn't immediately shame me about my flossing habits." That moment stuck with her all these years, and it was the reason she liked and trusted me from the start. Now, you might think that's a small thing — but it's not. The way we connect, engage, and communicate — even about something as seemingly benign as flossing — can leave a lasting imprint.

It's not about ignoring important issues or sugar-coating health advice to avoid offence. It's about *how* we deliver the message — choosing empathy over ego. My patients feel safe telling me the truth because they know they won't be met with judgment or criticism but with understanding instead. And that psychological safety is the foundation of real, honest, and effective healthcare.

By building trust and rapport through light-hearted interactions, we create a space where patients feel comfortable being completely honest about their habits and behaviours. This openness allows us to work together collaboratively, developing realistic solutions that support long-term health outcomes. In this way, empathetic engagement therefore not only enhances patient satisfaction but also contributes to a deeper sense of fulfilment in our work. The act of providing care that acknowledges and addresses the emotional as well as physical aspects of health reinforces the core values of the medical profession, strengthening the bond between patient and provider and satisfying our desire to help others, which is why most of us entered a medical profession in the first place.

EMPATHY AT WORK: THE RIPPLE EFFECT ON CULTURE AND WELLBEING

The cultivation of empathy within healthcare settings also has broader implications for the healthcare system as a whole. Teams characterised by high levels of empathetic understanding among members display greater collaboration, reduced conflict, and improved morale. These positive team dynamics don't just improve patient care and practice success — they also profoundly impact the daily experience of healthcare professionals, leading to a more fulfilling and less stressful work environment.

Considering the sheer amount of time we spend at work, the environment we create within our teams directly influences our overall quality of life and happiness. A workplace where empathy is embedded into daily interactions fosters a sense of psychological safety, where team members feel valued, supported, and respected. When people feel heard and understood, they are more likely to engage meaningfully with their work, experience higher job satisfaction, and develop a stronger sense of purpose. This, in turn, reduces stress, burnout, and emotional exhaustion — common challenges in healthcare that can otherwise take a significant toll on both professional and personal well-being.

Importantly, a positive work culture built on mutual respect and empathy extends beyond the walls of the workplace. The emotional weight of a toxic or stressful work environment doesn't stay at the office — it follows people home, affecting their mood, relationships with friends and family, and overall mental health. On the other hand, when work is a place of connection, teamwork, and shared purpose, that energy spills over into life outside of work. Healthcare professionals who feel supported and valued in their workplace are more likely to experience lower stress levels, better work-life balance, and a greater overall sense of happiness.

1.6 Stress and the Brain: Safeguarding Emotional Intelligence in the Face of Pressure

---

"It's not stress that kills us, it is our reaction to it."

— Hans Selye

Stress is more than just a feeling — it's a force that reshapes the emotional architecture of the brain. By understanding how stress impacts the emotional centres of the brain, we gain the power to recognise early warning signs so that we can build the habits and strategies that safeguard our empathy, regulate our reactions, and allow us to continue showing up as the calm, compassionate professionals our patients need.

In the demanding environment of healthcare, stress is as pervasive as the air we breathe, looming over even the most routine tasks, particularly in the early stages of our careers. Under this constant pressure, we can find ourselves grappling not just with the physical toll of our roles but with a continual threat of breakdown of our cognitive faculties which are crucial for emotional intelligence. This degradation leads to overwhelm, panic and an inability to think clearly so therefore manifests most acutely in the areas of emotional regulation and empathy, which as we now know are paramount for excellent patient care and continued professional satisfaction. The science examining the impact of stress on these cognitive functions paints a picture of a brain under siege, where the flood of stress hormones such as cortisol disrupts the delicate neural pathways responsible for processing and responding to emotional stimuli appropriately.

WHEN STRESS HIJACKS EMPATHY AND EMOTIONAL REGULATION

Under normal circumstances, the brain's prefrontal cortex acts as a moderating force, regulating emotional responses in a manner that allows for reasoned decision-making and empathetic engagement. However, under the relentless bombardment of stress, this regulatory capacity diminishes over time. Neural circuits become overwrought, leading to a state where emotional reactions are not tempered by rational thought but are instead experienced with heightened intensity and diminished control. This shift not only undermines our ability to engage empathetically with patients and make rational decisions but also impairs our capacity to manage our own emotional responses to the myriad stressors inherent in our work, leading to discontent and ultimately, burnout.

HOW CHRONIC STRESS DULLS EMPATHY IN THE BRAIN

Compounding this challenge is the impact of chronic stress on the brain's capacity for empathy. Empathy, the ability to understand and share the feelings of another, relies on a network of brain regions including the mirror neuron system we discussed earlier and the insula. These areas allow individuals to not just perceive but to viscerally experience the emotions of those around them. The insula, a small but powerful structure tucked deep within the cerebral cortex, plays a crucial role in processing emotions, bodily awareness, and interoception — the sense of what's happening within our own body. It acts as a bridge between our cognitive and emotional experiences, helping us tune into our own feelings and, crucially, allowing us to recognise and share in the emotions of others. In essence, the insula acts as the brain's empathy hub, helping us "feel" what someone else is going through, whether it's pain, joy, or distress.

However, chronic stress impairs the functionality of these brain regions. High levels of cortisol, the body's primary stress hormone, impair the insula's ability to accurately process emotional and physical sensations, dulling our empathetic acuity. Over time, this leads to empathy fatigue, where healthcare professionals become increasingly detached, emotionally numb, or even indifferent to patient suffering. Essentially, stress dulls the brain's ability to "tune in" to patients, making it harder to engage in meaningful, compassionate interactions. This reduced capacity to connect with patients on an emotional level can start to wear down the foundation of trust and understanding upon which effective patient care is built.

PROTECTING EMOTIONAL INTELLIGENCE THROUGH DAILY PRACTICE

Confronted with these challenges, it becomes imperative for us to adopt strategies aimed at mitigating the impact of stress on our emotional intelligence. Foremost among these strategies are techniques for stress management, designed to temper the physiological and psychological responses to stress. Mindfulness meditation, with its emphasis on present-moment awareness, offers a potent antidote to the mind's tendency to become caught up in a loop of stress-induced rumination. By fostering a state of detached observation, we can gain perspective on our stressors, reducing their emotional intensity and reclaiming a measure of control over our responses.

Similarly, physical exercise can be used as a powerful tool for stress reduction. Beyond its well-documented benefits for physical health, regular exercise induces a cascade of neurochemical changes that counteract the effects of stress. Endorphins, often dubbed the brain's "feel-good" neurotransmitters, are released during physical activity, providing a natural mood lift that can alleviate the burden of stress. Exercise also promotes neurogenesis in the hippocampus, a brain region integral to stress and mood regulation and emotional processing. This improved neural connectivity can lead to better stress resilience, enhanced emotional well-being, and overall cognitive flexibility, highlighting the profound impact of physical activity on brain health and emotional resilience.

Taking a walk outdoors, whether in the early morning to set the tone for the day or during a lunch break to reset, can be a simple yet profoundly effective way to manage stress and enhance emotional well-being. Time spent in nature has been shown to lower cortisol levels, reduce anxiety, and improve mood, making it a powerful antidote to the pressures of a demanding healthcare career. A concept known as "forest bathing" (or Shinrin-yoku in Japanese) emphasises the therapeutic benefits of immersing oneself in a natural environment. Simply being among trees, breathing in fresh air, and absorbing the sights and sounds of nature can calm the nervous system, enhance focus, and even boost immune function. Even if a full forest is not accessible, walking through a park, by a body of water, or anywhere with greenery can provide similar grounding effects. These mindful moments of connection with nature can help us to recharge, regain perspective, and cultivate emotional balance, ultimately allowing us to return to our work with greater clarity and resilience.

Equally important is the cultivation of social support networks within the healthcare environment. This can include local study clubs or even groups on social media apps such as Facebook. The act of sharing experiences and challenges with colleagues creates a buffer against the isolating effects of stress. These connections provide not just emotional solace but also practical strategies for managing stress, fostering a communal resilience that can bolster individual efforts. Through peer support, we can create a culture of mutual care and understanding, reinforcing the emotional bonds that underpin effective teamwork and patient care.

Healthcare organisations, both large institutions and small businesses, have a crucial role in supporting the emotional well-being of their teams. In larger organisations, structured programs — such as stress management workshops, mindfulness training, and group fitness classes — can provide healthcare professionals and their teams with practical tools to manage the pressures of their roles. These initiatives not only help prevent burnout and compassion fatigue, but they also send a clear message that the institution values its team members as people first, not just professionals.

While large hospitals and healthcare networks often have the resources to implement these kinds of programs on a broad scale, small businesses, including private practices, can incorporate similar principles in more personalised ways. Simple changes — like encouraging regular breaks, promoting a culture of open communication, or scheduling occasional team wellness and bonding activities — can create an environment where emotional well-being is prioritised. Even something as straightforward as a weekly check-in with staff to discuss stress levels and workload can make a significant difference.

Chapter 2

Connecting with Patients Through Emotional Intelligence

2.1 Building Rapport from the First Interaction

> *"Rapport is the ability to enter someone else's world, to make him feel that you understand him, that you have a strong common bond."*
>
> — Tony Robbins

WHY FIRST IMPRESSIONS MATTER

The connection between a patient and their provider sets the tone for the entire framework of care. This foundational connection, best known as rapport, transcends mere pleasantries, instead embodying a profound understanding and mutual respect that significantly influences the trajectory of healthcare delivery. I cannot emphasise enough the importance of establishing a strong connection between healthcare providers and patients, particularly in the context of dentistry where long-term care is the goal and therefore establishing and maintaining trust over time is pivotal. It is key to remember that it is in the initial moments of interaction that patients gauge their safety and belonging within the healthcare environment, determining their willingness to divulge concerns, adhere to proposed treatments, and engage actively in their care journey.

THE POWER OF PRESENCE AND CLEAR COMMUNICATION

Establishing clear and transparent communication channels fosters openness and encourages patients to express their needs and preferences freely. Additionally, showing respect for patients' autonomy and involving them in decision-making processes cultivates a sense of partnership and empowerment.

One of the simplest yet most powerful tools in building this kind of connection is using a patient's name. As Dale Carnegie famously said, *"A person's name is to that person, the sweetest, most important sound in any language."* Remembering and using someone's name communicates respect, recognition, and personal attention. It reinforces that they are not just another appointment or chart number, but a unique individual who matters. This small gesture can have a big impact — quickly building rapport, helping patients feel seen and valued, and strengthening trust from the very first interaction.

Building an authentic connection requires an intentional presence, a conscious effort to be fully with the patient, not just in the physical space but mentally and emotionally attuned to their experiences and needs. This presence, a hallmark of emotional intelligence, fosters an environment where trust flourishes and openness becomes the norm.

One of the most effective ways to invite this openness is by asking open-ended questions — questions that go beyond yes-or-no answers and encourage patients to share more of their story. These types of questions help us better understand what matters to the person in front of us, not just their health condition or symptoms. When patients feel genuinely heard, they're more likely to relax, engage, and reveal the deeper context that might otherwise go unnoticed. And in those moments of sharing, we're given valuable opportunities to find common ground and build connection.

Instead of defaulting to generic or surface-level questions like "How are you today?" or "What do you do for work?", consider asking something that invites a more personal, positive response. For example:

- "What's something exciting or interesting going on in your life right now?"
- "What are your favourite things to do on the weekend?"
- "What's a goal you're working on at the moment?"
- "Are you planning anything fun or relaxing this week/weekend?"
- "What's something that's been bringing you joy lately?"
- "What's new with you?"

These types of questions give patients permission to talk about their passions, priorities, and personalities — not just their problems. They not only spark richer conversation but also subtly shift the tone of the interaction from clinical to human, building warmth and trust from the very start.

THE POWER OF SINCERE COMPLIMENTS

Compliments — when offered sincerely — are a powerful and often underused way to build rapport. But not all compliments are created equal. Generic praise like "I like your jumper" may land flat or feel impersonal. In contrast, a well-justified compliment not only feels more genuine but activates the right side of the brain — the creative, emotional, relational part that fosters connection. For example: "Wow, I love that colour on you — it really makes your eyes pop!" This kind of specific and personal compliment is more likely to be received as authentic, helping the patient feel seen and appreciated.

Compliments can also help us reframe potentially negative situations that might otherwise damage rapport. Imagine the difference between:

- "Sorry I'm running late, we're short-staffed today..."

vs.

- "We're short-staffed today — thank you so much for your patience."

The first focuses on the inconvenience. The second turns the same situation into a moment of appreciation, helping patients feel respected rather than neglected.

These small shifts in language do more than soften interactions — they build emotional bridges. Sincere compliments, especially when unexpected or delivered with presence, can set the tone for trust, defuse tension, and turn routine care into a relationship.

FINDING COMMON GROUND

During my final year of dental school, I ventured to a rural town for my very first interview for a dental position. The interview panel consisted of the practice owner and her father, who happened to be a lawyer. After the standard interview questions, the owner's father unexpectedly inquired if I played golf. I admitted that I didn't, to which he responded, "Well, how will you connect with your patients if you don't play golf?" I was taken aback by the absurdity of the question. It left a lasting impression on me because it seemed so out of touch. However, it underscored the importance of shared experiences in building rapport. While it may have seemed like everyone in that town was a golf enthusiast, it highlighted the value of finding common ground with our patients.

The difference is, we don't have to *guess* what that common ground might be — we can simply ask. By engaging patients with curiosity, listening actively, and sharing aspects of our own humanity, we uncover meaningful connections that transform routine care into a truly relational experience.

BEYOND THE FIRST ENCOUNTER: RELIABILITY AND FOLLOW-THROUGH

Importantly, rapport-building extends far beyond the initial encounter, necessitating consistent reinforcement through every phase of care and by each member of the team — not just the clinician. Beyond interpersonal skills, consistency, reliability, and follow-through in care delivery are the glue that holds the relationship together over time. When healthcare providers and team members do what they say they will — whether it's calling with results, checking in on a patient's progress, or simply being on time — it communicates respect and builds a sense of psychological safety. Patients learn that they can count on you. In contrast, broken promises, long delays, or missed details can chip away at trust, even if the intentions are good. In a busy healthcare environment, reliability becomes a quiet form of empathy: showing up consistently sends the message that your patient's wellbeing is a priority, not just in words, but in action. It's these moments of follow-through that build lasting rapport based on mutual respect and understanding.

VERBAL AND NON-VERBAL COMMUNICATION

Building rapport with our patients is an artful blend of empathy, communication, and trust-building. As discussed, it begins with active listening, where healthcare providers engage attentively with patients, validating their concerns and demonstrating genuine interest in their well-being. Empathetic responses, conveyed through both verbal and nonverbal cues, help patients feel understood and respected.

A tidy trio of numbers — 7, 38, 55 — helps explain just how powerful these cues can be: only 7% of an emotional message is communicated through the actual words we speak, while 38% is conveyed through tone of voice and a striking 55% through body language. These figures, derived from psychologist Albert Mehrabian's communication theory, highlight the critical role of nonverbal communication in conveying empathy and emotion. This is why techniques for swiftly establishing rapport often pivot on non-verbal communication. A genuine smile, the subtle forward lean of engagement, and the maintenance of appropriate eye contact serve as silent signs of empathy and attentiveness. These unspoken signals, when paired with thoughtful verbal communication, create a harmonious interaction that reassures patients of their value and individuality. Body language and non-verbal cues will be explored further in Section 2.4.

SETTING THE SCENE: PHYSICAL ENVIRONMENT AND SENSORY IMPACT

Attention should also be paid to the physical environment also as this extends beyond mere aesthetics and plays a role in rapport-building, and therefore strong consideration should be given to privacy, comfort, and an atmosphere free from distractions, underscoring a commitment to relationship-centred care. For instance, ensuring ample privacy during consultations fosters an environment where patients feel safe to openly discuss their concerns and preferences. Comfortable seating arrangements and soothing decor contribute to a sense of ease and relaxation, facilitating more meaningful interactions. Minimising noise and distractions within the clinical setting allows patients to focus on the conversation at hand, enhancing their overall experience and reinforcing the notion of relationship-centred care. In addition, incorporating calming scents through the use of candles or essential oil diffusers can further enhance the patient experience, promoting a soothing atmosphere conducive to rapport-building and relaxation. This is particularly important in dentistry where the smell of latex and chemicals can be overwhelming and sometimes even triggering for some patients.

Just the other day, I had a new patient come in for her first appointment. She was noticeably anxious and mentioned she'd been dreading the visit for days. But as she walked into our reception area, she paused and commented on how nice it smelled. She said the calming scent immediately helped her feel more at ease, even before speaking to anyone. It was a simple detail, but it genuinely shifted her mindset and made her feel more comfortable. It's these small, sensory touches that can be easily dismissed or overlooked as irrelevant but can have a powerful impact — especially for anxious patients — and further reinforce that they're in a safe, caring space.

THE ROLE OF TRUST IN PATIENT RELATIONSHIPS

There is a symbiotic relationship between rapport and trust which serves as the bedrock for effective healthcare delivery. Trust, in this context, goes beyond the belief in the healthcare professional's competence, instead encompassing faith in their empathy, confidentiality, and commitment to the patient's best interest. This trust paves the way for a collaborative partnership, where patients feel empowered to take an active role in their care, confident in the support and guidance of their healthcare provider. The resultant openness not only enriches the quality of information shared but also enhances our ability to tailor care to our patient's unique circumstances, preferences, and values.

Our role is to support our patients in whatever level of care they decide is right for them without judgment, recognising that everyone's journey towards wellness is deeply personal and subjective. By fostering an environment of acceptance and understanding, we empower our patients to make informed decisions about their health, respecting their autonomy and dignity every step of the way.

THE POWER OF RAPPORT IN HEALTH OUTCOMES

Further, the impact of rapport on health outcomes cannot be overstated. Studies have consistently shown that strong patient-provider relationships, characterised by mutual respect and understanding, significantly contribute to improved health behaviours, treatment adherence, and overall satisfaction with care. Patients who feel understood and supported are more likely to follow through with recommended treatments, engage in proactive health behaviours, and participate in decision-making processes. Also, the positive emotional state fostered by effective rapport can itself be therapeutic, contributing to an enhanced sense of well-being and, in some cases, influencing physiological responses to treatment. That is, it has a profound effect on the mental and mindset component of healing.

Research in psychoneuroimmunology suggests that our mental state and mindset can significantly impact our physiological responses to treatment and recovery. When patients feel understood, supported, and valued by their healthcare providers, it can trigger a cascade of beneficial effects in the brain and body. Positive emotions such as hope, optimism, and trust have been linked to improved immune function, reduced levels of stress hormones, and enhanced resilience in the face of illness. Moreover, cultivating a mindset of resilience and active engagement in one's healing process has been shown to positively influence treatment outcomes and recovery trajectories.

I saw this firsthand during my time working as a pharmacy assistant in a small, community pharmacy while studying at university. Many of the customers were regulars who had been coming in for years, and over time, we got to know them incredibly well — their routines, their stories, their quirks, and even their families. It struck me how often two people with seemingly similar conditions could have such vastly different experiences, simply based on their outlook. Patients who approached their health with optimism and a proactive mindset often reported fewer symptoms, recovered more quickly, and generally coped better overall. In contrast, those who felt hopeless or defeated by their diagnosis often seemed to struggle more — not just emotionally, but physically as well. It was a powerful early lesson in the connection between mindset and medicine. By nurturing a therapeutic alliance built on empathy, trust, and mutual respect, we as healthcare providers not only enhance the patient experience but also harness the powerful interplay between mind and body to promote healing and well-being.

RECONSIDERING TITLES: PROFESSIONALISM VS RELATABILITY

Another important yet often overlooked aspect of rapport building is how we use professional titles — particularly the title "Doctor" — when interacting with patients. While this is standard practice in places like the United States, where professional formality is deeply ingrained in the culture, here in Australia we tend to have a more relaxed and down-to-earth approach. Personally, I've found that strictly enforcing the use of the doctor title can create unnecessary distance between us and our patients. It reinforces a sense of hierarchy, making our interactions feel less like conversations and more like lectures. In my view, insisting on being called "Doctor" at all times is more about ego than professionalism. Our patients know we're qualified — there's no need to keep reminding them. That said, I understand that some worry it might cross a professional boundary to be too casual, and this is a valid concern. But I believe it's possible to drop our guard and be relatable without compromising professionalism. For instance, I always introduce myself to patients simply as "Lora," but I ensure that my team consistently refers to me as "Dr Lora" when speaking about me in front of patients. This strikes a balance that helps to build trust while maintaining professional respect. I once worked with a colleague who had spent years practicing in the U.S. before moving to Australia. She was shocked — and even brought to tears — the first time a team member here used her first name in front of a patient. Back in the States, other team members didn't even know her first name. However, I truly believe that when you have confidence in your abilities and value your contribution, you don't need to hide behind titles. True professionalism isn't about what people call you — it's about how you make them feel.

HUMOUR: A SURPRISING BRIDGE TO CONNECTION

Humour is one of the most underutilised yet powerful tools we have at our disposal. It has the potential to disarm anxiety, create connection, and shift the tone of even the most challenging interactions. In my own practice, I use humour daily — whether it's a light-hearted comment or a cheeky observation — as a way to build rapport, put patients at ease, and create a more human, relaxed environment. I've found that even a small, well-timed joke can release tension in the room, making a nervous patient feel seen, safe, and understood. It's not about being a stand-up comedian or undermining the seriousness of a situation — it's about knowing when and how to use humour to strengthen the therapeutic relationship.

The research backs this up. Studies have shown that humour, when used appropriately, can enhance communication, reduce patient stress, and improve satisfaction. In fact, humour has been described as a "social lubricant," helping to smooth interpersonal interactions and make clinicians appear more relatable. The presence of laughter can foster a sense of equality between clinician and patient, breaking down the perceived hierarchy that often exists in clinical settings. This levelling effect can be particularly important in environments like dentistry, where patients may feel vulnerable or apprehensive. What's more, laughter triggers the release of endorphins — the body's natural feel-good chemicals — which help to ease tension, reduce anxiety, and create a more relaxed, positive atmosphere for both patient and practitioner. When I share a laugh with a patient — even if it's just about the eternal mystery of whether anyone *actually* flosses daily — it creates a sense of camaraderie that carries through the entire appointment.

One of my favourite examples of this comes from a regular patient who came in for his six-month check-up at 8am on a Saturday morning. As he settled into the chair and I joked about him getting up so early just to see the dentist, he laughed and said, "You know, it's not fun to go to the dentist... well, it kind of is." It caught me off guard in the best way. What he meant, of course, was that although nobody *loves* coming to the dentist, our appointments had become something he didn't dread — because we always shared a laugh. It was a light-hearted comment, but for me, it spoke volumes. It was a reminder that humour has the power to completely shift how people experience care. Something as small as making someone laugh or helping them feel at ease can change their entire relationship with healthcare — from something they avoid, to something they're actually happy to return to.

Of course, humour in healthcare is not without its risks. It can easily backfire if it's misjudged or poorly timed, especially in emotionally charged or sensitive situations. It requires emotional intelligence to gauge the mood of the room, understand the individual sitting across from you, and assess what type of humour — if any — is appropriate. There are also cultural and personal factors to consider. What one patient finds hilarious, another might find offensive or confusing. This is where empathy and awareness become crucial. Humour should always be patient-centred. It should never be used to mask discomfort, make light of a patient's concerns, or centre ourselves in the interaction. Instead, it should serve as a bridge — something that connects, rather than divides.

Importantly, humour isn't just for the patient's benefit — it also plays a critical role in clinician wellbeing. Healthcare is emotionally demanding, and the constant exposure to stress, suffering, and high-stakes decision-making can take its toll. Humour acts as a pressure valve. It gives us, as clinicians, a way to cope, to decompress, and to stay connected to the joy and humanity in our work. Shared laughter with colleagues can lighten the emotional load and create a sense of camaraderie in teams, helping us get through long, demanding days. Research even shows that humour may buffer against burnout and compassion fatigue by fostering resilience and emotional regulation.

I was recently chatting with someone I met at a business conference — she had previously worked as a nurse in both emergency and paediatric oncology. As we spoke about her career, she shared that developing a sense of dark humour was essential for her survival in those roles. "Some of the things I saw were just so awful," she told me. "You either cry, or you laugh — and sometimes, laughter was the only thing that helped us get through it." Her words stuck with me. They were a powerful reminder that humour, even when dark, is not about dismissing pain — it's often about finding a lifeline in the midst of it. It's a way to stay human in environments where the emotional weight can feel unbearable.

This is exactly why one of the most powerful aspects of humour is its ability to humanise us. Patients often enter healthcare settings expecting a certain level of formality or detachment. But when we let our guard down — even slightly — with a joke or a playful remark, we remind them that we're human too. That we care. This humanisation helps build trust. It reassures patients that they're not just another appointment in a packed schedule — they're being seen and cared for by someone who genuinely connects with them as a whole person.

In many ways, humour is an extension of empathy. It's a way of saying, "I see you, I get you, and I'm here with you." Like any tool, it needs to be used with care and good judgement — but when used thoughtfully, humour can create lasting impressions and deepen the therapeutic alliance. In a field where we deal daily with fear, uncertainty, and sometimes grief, humour reminds us all — patients and clinicians alike — that healing is not only about what we do, but how we connect with each other along the way.

WHY RAPPORT STILL MATTERS IN A TECHNOLOGICAL AGE

In the ever-evolving landscape of healthcare technology, the enduring importance of rapport in patient care remains constant. It serves as a powerful reminder that even as innovations transform the way we diagnose and treat, the heart of healthcare is still deeply human — driven by connections that comfort, empower, and heal. In today's increasingly competitive healthcare environment, this truth holds greater weight than ever. For clinicians committed to delivering exceptional care, cultivating strong rapport is not just an indispensable skill — it is a foundational element of both the art and science of healing.

2.2 Principles of Emotionally Intelligent Communication

> *"It is very important to understand that emotional intelligence is not the opposite of intelligence, it is not the triumph of heart over head – it is the unique intersection of both."*
>
> — David Caruso

Once rapport has been initiated, it's the quality of our communication that maintains and deepens the connection. Emotionally intelligent communication is the vehicle through which trust, understanding, and collaboration are strengthened. At the core of effective communication in healthcare lies a set of guiding principles — clarity, active listening, respect, and confidentiality — each serving as a pillar that supports the bridge between providers and those we serve.

Clarity ensures messages are understood as intended, free from the fog of medical jargon or ambiguity. It is critical to master the skill of using layman's terms to convey the patient's medical condition and associated treatment options to the patient. I believe that the use of medical jargon only serves to inflate the ego and create a power differential between the health professional and the patient which is counterproductive to establishing an open and collaborative partnership. With any professional, and this is not exclusive to healthcare, there will exist a knowledge gap between the professional and the layman. The responsibility of the professional is to bridge the knowledge gap just enough for the patient to clearly understand their condition and options, enabling informed consent — without overwhelming them. After all, the patient is there to see you for your expertise. They are aware of the qualifications that you hold. They understand that you have the knowledge and skills required for the profession that you are practicing in, otherwise, you would not be there. Therefore, maintaining a conversation purely based in medical jargon does nothing except wedge a gap between the professional and patient and does not empower the patient to take control of their own situation and the care they need, nor does it help to build trust and rapport.

Active listening fosters a space where patients and colleagues feel heard, validating their experiences and concerns. By employing active listening, we can demonstrate empathy and respect, which can strengthen the therapeutic alliance and enhance the satisfaction our patients feel with the level of care that we provide. This practice not only promotes trust and rapport but also allows for a deeper understanding of our patients' needs and preferences, leading to more personalised and effective care interventions.

Respect must underpin every interaction, acknowledging the dignity and worth of every individual regardless of their health status or role within the healthcare system. We are not any better than our patients because we have a medical degree, we simply have the necessary specific training to provide the health services that they need and should approach our interactions with this attitude of empathy and humility at the forefront of our minds. If we do this, we can foster a culture of mutual respect and collaboration, ultimately enhancing the quality of care and patient outcomes.

Finally, confidentiality safeguards the trust placed in us as health-care professionals, protecting the intimate details shared in vulnerable moments but also upholds ethical standards and legal obligations. By safeguarding the privacy of our patients' sensitive information, we demonstrate our commitment to respecting autonomy and fostering a safe and supportive environment for open communication and care.

FROM UNDERSTANDING TO CONNECTION

Empathy in communication goes beyond mere understanding; it involves feeling with the patient, stepping into their shoes to grasp the emotional undertones of their words. Techniques that can be used to infuse empathy into communication include reflective listening, where the healthcare professional mirrors the patient's feelings, acknowledging their emotions and concerns. Another method involves using empathetic statements that explicitly acknowledge the patient's perspective, such as "It sounds like this has been a really tough time for you," which serves to validate their feelings and build rapport. These techniques and others will be discussed in more detail in Section 2.3.

STEPPING IN THEIR WORLD: THE POWER OF THE EMPATHY MAP

To further explore the concept of empathy in healthcare communication, we can consider the use of an "Empathy Map." This visual tool can help us delve deeper into the patient's experience, encouraging reflection on what the patient might be thinking, feeling, hearing, and seeing. By filling out an Empathy Map, we can gain a more holistic view of the patient's world, aiding in the development of more empathetic communication strategies.

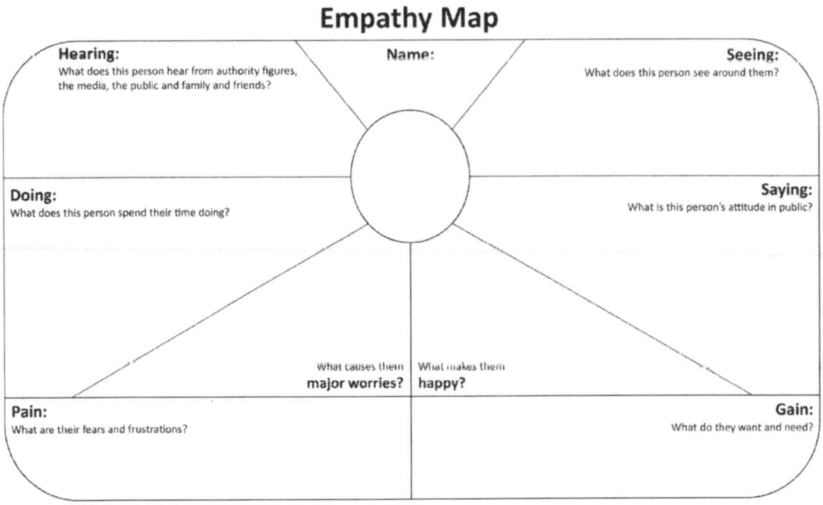

A study conducted by Cairns et. al in the UK, published in 2020, states that "Empathy is a cornerstone of patient-centred care. However, empathy levels among health care professionals and medical students are currently suboptimal. An empathy map is a tool which aids in understanding another person's perspective. Empathy maps have up until now not been used in a medical education setting." The article explores the application of empathy mapping in medical education to enhance students' understanding of patients' experiences and perspectives. It introduces a novel approach called the "medical empathy map," which provides a structured framework for students to analyse patients' emotions, thoughts, and behaviours. The map includes four quadrants focusing on patients' feelings, concerns, goals, and influencing factors. It explains that by engaging in empathy mapping exercises, students develop a deeper appreciation for the complex interplay of factors shaping our patients' experiences, ultimately improving their ability to deliver patient-centred care. The study highlights the efficacy of empathy mapping in fostering empathy, communication skills, and patient-centeredness among medical students, suggesting its potential as a valuable tool in medical education curriculum. This idea can be applied across all health professions and extend beyond students into professionals as well.

BEYOND THE WORDS WE USE

Non-verbal cues, from facial expressions and body posture to the subtleties of eye contact, play a significant role in healthcare communication. These silent signals can reinforce the words that we speak, conveying empathy, concern, and attentiveness. For instance, a simple act like sitting down to talk to a patient at eye level instead of standing over them can powerfully communicate care and presence, making the patient feel valued and respected. Similarly, being mindful of one's own body language, ensuring it is open and inviting, can significantly enhance the quality of interactions, fostering an environment of trust and openness. It is also important that we learn to read our patient's body language to ensure the words they are speaking to us match the signals their body is sending us. For example, during a treatment session, if we inquire about the patient's well-being and they verbally confirm they are fine, but we observe tightly clasped hands and rapid breathing, it's crucial to recognise this incongruence between their words and body language. In such instances, it's essential to pause or halt the treatment to ensure the patient's comfort and address any unmet needs promptly. We will discuss non-verbal cues and body language in more detail in Section 2.4.

GRACE UNDER PRESSURE: COMMUNICATING WITH COMPASSION IN CHALLENGING MOMENTS

Discussing sensitive health issues or delivering bad news is an inevitable aspect of healthcare that requires not just tact but a profound sense of empathy and ethical consideration. Strategies for these conversations include preparation, taking the time to gather all necessary information and anticipating patient questions. Setting a compassionate tone from the outset, ensuring privacy, and using clear, straightforward language can help navigate these conversations with dignity and respect. It is also vital to offer support and resources, guiding patients and families toward understanding and acceptance. This will be discussed in more detail in Section 2.6.

Whether we're speaking, listening, or simply present in the room, how we communicate shapes every aspect of patient care. In every patient interaction lies the potential for healing beyond the physical, reaching into the realms of emotional and psychological well-being. By mastering the art and science of communication, healthcare professionals unlock the door to more meaningful patient relationships, improved care outcomes, and a more fulfilling professional experience. This chapter serves as a guide for those committed to transforming healthcare interactions through the power of emotional intelligence, fostering an environment where every word, every gesture, and every pause speaks volumes. Now, let's dive right in!

2.3 Listening to Understand: The True Power of Presence

> *"I had listened intently. I had listened because I was genuinely interested. And he felt it. Naturally that pleased him. That kind of listening is one of the highest compliments we can pay anyone."*
>
> — Dale Carnegie

Listening might sound simple, but when you truly do it with empathy, it becomes an entirely different skillset — one that takes intention and practice. Empathetic listening isn't just about hearing the words someone says. It's about being fully present, whether with a patient, a colleague, or a member of your wider team. Across every touchpoint in healthcare — whether clinician to patient or team member to team member — deep listening fosters connection, trust, and collaboration. It means paying attention to the bigger picture — what's going on in this person's life that might be influencing how they're feeling or what they're telling you today?

When we listen in this way, we're not rushing to respond or jumping in with a solution the moment there's a pause. Instead, we're holding space. We're allowing the patient to feel heard and understood, which is incredibly powerful. Our responses become less about fixing and more about validating — letting the patient know that their experience matters and that we're here to support them, not just clinically, but as a human being.

This kind of listening builds trust, breaks down barriers, and sets the stage for meaningful connection. It might take a little more time, but the payoff in patient cooperation, satisfaction, and overall outcomes is worth it. As Ernest Hemingway once wrote, *"When people talk, listen completely. Most people never listen."* This quote captures the gap between simply hearing and truly listening — something that, in healthcare, can mark the difference between a transactional exchange and a transformative connection. It's a powerful reminder that while listening may appear passive, doing it well requires presence, intention, and genuine care. It's such a vital part of emotionally intelligent practice that we'll be diving deeper into it in this section.

CREATING A SAFE SPACE FOR SHARING

Crafting an environment conducive to open dialogue and uninhibited sharing demands more than physical comfort; it necessitates an atmosphere that provides an air of psychological safety. This level of security is not garnered through grand gestures but through the subtleties of genuine concern, patience, and the unwavering presence of the listener. Such a space invites our patients to unveil their fears, hopes, and pain, secure in the knowledge that their words will be met with empathy and understanding from us as their healthcare providers. This process needs to begin with the deliberate removal of barriers — both literal, such as a physical layout that might intimidate, and figurative, represented by our demeanour, language, and approachability. We should always aim to adopt a demeanour that exudes warmth, empathy, and approachability, as this is likely to reassure patients and make them feel comfortable opening up to us about their concerns. I have had patients feel comfortable enough to tell me all sorts of personal information (often unrelated to their dental health), ranging from their family struggles to their anxieties about upcoming procedures. These moments of openness underscore the importance of cultivating an environment where patients feel safe and supported, enabling them to share their dental concerns and broader life experiences. This holistic approach to patient care fosters trust, strengthens the patient-provider relationship, and ultimately enhances the overall quality of care delivered.

THE CONSEQUENCES OF COMMUNICATION BREAKDOWN

Language plays a crucial role as well; using clear, jargon-free communication and mindfully listening to patients without judgment or interruption can break down barriers to honest dialogue. Using layman's terms when discussing medical issues with patients is crucial for ensuring understanding and empowerment. Failing to do so can lead to confusion, anxiety, and a sense of disempowerment, ultimately hindering effective communication and shared decision-making in healthcare. Let's consider the following scenario:

During a routine dental check-up, Dr Dentist explained to Mr Patient that he had "large distal-occlusal caries close to the pulp on the upper left second molar" that required treatment. Mr Patient, unfamiliar with dental terminology, nodded along, feeling somewhat puzzled. As Dr Dentist proceeded to explain the various treatment options using more technical language, Mr Patient's confusion deepened. He couldn't decipher whether he needed a simple filling or a more extensive procedure. Feeling overwhelmed and unsure, Mr Patient hesitated to make a decision. He left the appointment feeling anxious and uncertain about his dental health.

In the following days, Mr Patient mulled over his options, but the jargon-laden explanation from Dr Dentist left him feeling frustrated and disconnected from the decision-making process. He even considered seeking a second opinion from another dentist to clarify his treatment options. Eventually, Mr Patient decided to delay the treatment until he could better understand the procedure and its implications.

What are the potential consequences in the above scenario? Whilst it may not seem like anything untoward has happened in the above scenario, the consequences of the patient and doctor failing to establish a connection and build trust are significant. For the patient, the lack of clarity regarding the necessary treatment has led to indecision and delayed care. Consequently, untreated dental issues can worsen over time, potentially necessitating more complex and costly treatments in the future. This not only impacts the patient's oral health but also their overall well-being and quality of life. For the dentist, the inability to effectively communicate treatment options and engage patients in decision-making may result in a loss of trust and confidence in their practice. This could lead to patient dissatisfaction, negative reviews, and ultimately, a decline in patient retention. Therefore, fostering effective patient-doctor communication is essential for ensuring optimal outcomes and maintaining a thriving dental practice. In the medical profession, the consequences of delaying treatment can be, and usually are, even more significant than this example in the dental setting.

SIMPLIFYING LANGUAGE & USING ANALOGIES

If he chooses to reflect on the experience, Dr Dentist could realise that his use of medical jargon had inadvertently hindered Mr Patient's ability to make an informed decision about his dental care. Determined to improve communication with his patients, Dr Dentist could make a conscious effort to simplify his explanations, using layman's terms to ensure clarity and understanding. In doing so, he will empower his patients to actively participate in their dental care decisions, fostering trust and confidence in their treatment journey.

One of the most effective ways to communicate complex information is by using analogies that patients can easily relate to. For example, when treating patients with gum disease who have no noticeable symptoms, I often liken the condition to termites eating away at the foundations of a house. You wouldn't invest in renovations — like whitening, cosmetic work, or orthodontics — if the structure underneath wasn't stable. In the same way, it's not wise to focus on restoring or improving the appearance of teeth if the bones and gums that support them aren't healthy.

Another example I often use is when a patient is deciding whether to save an infected tooth with root canal treatment or remove it altogether. I explain that taking out a tooth is like pulling a book from a fully packed bookshelf — doing so creates a gap that often leads to tipping, drifting, and bite problems later on. These simple visual comparisons help patients see the bigger picture and understand the long-term impact of their choices.

These are just two examples from dentistry, but the same approach can be used across all healthcare disciplines. Clinicians from different fields can brainstorm analogies that resonate with their patient base and use them to explain complex procedures, diagnoses, or treatment pathways. These explanations don't just make the information more accessible — they show patients that we care enough to meet them where they're at. That's when real trust is built.

POWERFUL QUESTIONING TECHNIQUES

To further improve clarity and communication, I've found it helpful to pause and ask the patient, "Does that make sense?" after explaining a condition or treatment plan. It gives them the space to process and reflect, and often prompts further questions or clarifications that might not have otherwise been raised. Even better, you can ask them to repeat back what they've understood in their own words — this not only reinforces their comprehension but gives you insight into any gaps that need to be addressed.

It's also worth considering switching the way we invite questions. Instead of asking, "Do you have any questions?" — which people often decline out of politeness or fear of seeming ignorant — try asking, "What questions do you have?" It's a subtle shift, but it opens the door and normalises curiosity, signalling that questions are expected and welcome. These small but powerful changes in communication — particularly converting closed questions to open-ended ones — layered with empathy and clear explanations, help create the kind of safe, respectful environment where patients feel heard, empowered, and genuinely cared for.

MASTERING VERBAL CUES: TONE, VOLUME & PACING

Ensuring we are approachable hinges not only on being non-judgmental and attentive to a patient's comfort, but also on adapting the pace and depth of our communication to meet them where they are emotionally. This means becoming skilled at interpreting both verbal and non-verbal cues and adjusting our delivery accordingly. Just as important as what we say is how we say it. Our tone of voice plays a powerful role in shaping how our message is received — capable of softening difficult conversations or, if misused, unintentionally adding tension to even neutral statements. A warm, steady tone can convey reassurance and empathy, while a rushed or clipped tone may be perceived as impatient or dismissive, even if that's not the intention. Likewise, speaking too quickly can overwhelm someone who is already anxious, whereas a calm, measured pace can help anchor and soothe them. Adjusting our volume is also important — raising our voice too much may feel intimidating, while speaking too softly could make a patient feel dismissed or unimportant. These vocal nuances are especially critical in emotionally charged or vulnerable moments when patients are often hyper-aware of our every word and gesture. Being mindful of our tone, volume, and pacing adds another layer of emotional intelligence to our communication, reinforcing that we are fully present and genuinely invested in the patient's experience.

Equally important is the mindset we bring into these interactions. Approaching every conversation with empathy and without judgment creates a safe space where patients feel respected and accepted, regardless of their circumstances or choices. This sense of psychological safety encourages honesty, vulnerability, and collaboration. Ultimately, cultivating a non-judgmental presence is foundational to building a therapeutic relationship rooted in mutual respect and trust — one that allows patients to engage fully and confidently in their care.

ACTIVE LISTENING IN PATIENT ASSESSMENT

At the intersection of diagnosis and empathy lies the critical role of active listening — a skill that elevates patient assessment from a routine examination to an insightful exploration of the individual's holistic health. Active listening transcends the passive reception of words, engaging with the patient's narrative to uncover layers of meaning often obscured by the superficial presentation of symptoms. This attentive listening facilitates a deeper understanding of not just the physiological symptoms but the emotional, social, and environmental factors contributing to the patient's condition. The key word here is understanding. In the words of Isaac F. Marcossen, "*They have been so much concerned with what they are going to say next that they do not keep their ears open...*". This is unfortunately very common and hinders the ability to establish trust and rapport with our patients. We must learn to listen to understand the patient fully, instead of simply to respond next with whatever it is that we are thinking.

As outlined in a Heart Matters Magazine article, active listening involves being fully present and engaged during conversations, allowing individuals to feel heard and understood. Practical strategies include maintaining eye contact, nodding to demonstrate understanding, and using verbal cues like "I see" or "Tell me more" to encourage further sharing. Another simple yet effective way to invite elaboration is by repeating the last word or a few key words the patient has said, but with an upward inflection that turns it into a gentle question. For example, if a patient says, "I've had such bad experiences with the dentist in the past," you might respond with, "Bad experiences?" This technique encourages them to expand on their thoughts in a way that feels natural and validating, without interrupting their flow. These small, intentional actions send a powerful message: I'm listening, and what you're saying matters. Patients also feel more connected to you when you use their own words back to them instead of rephrasing them — it's a subtle way of saying, "I hear you," and helps build trust because you're meeting them where they are, not pulling them into your world. When it comes to eye contact during a conversation, it's essential to strike the right balance. Since excessive eye contact can feel intimidating, adjusting it based on the situation is key. To demonstrate active listening without overwhelming the other person, try breaking eye contact every few seconds. Another effective technique is to alternate your gaze between their eyes and their mouth, spending about five seconds on each. When you do look away, it's best to glance to the side or up, as looking down might convey disinterest in continuing the conversation.

Importantly, active listening entails refraining from interrupting and reflecting back what has been heard to ensure accuracy and validation. Being interrupted can be incredibly frustrating for the other person, as it may convey a sense of superiority or a lack of interest in what they have to say. If you tend to be a quick thinker or speaker, make a conscious effort to slow down to allow the other person ample time to express themselves. Remember, it's okay to embrace moments of silence without feeling the need to interject. Allowing the other person to speak not only demonstrates respect but also facilitates better understanding of their message. Even well-intentioned interruptions, such as responding to something they've said, can derail the conversation from its original course. If this occurs, gently guide the conversation back on track by refocusing on what they were sharing. When emotions start to bubble up in response to what you're hearing, it can cloud your ability to fully engage with what comes next. Stay committed to active listening, and resist the temptation to anticipate what the speaker will say next.

If you're struggling to stay tuned in to the conversation, a helpful tactic is to silently repeat the speaker's words in your mind as they speak. This not only reinforces their message but also aids in maintaining focus. Additionally, it's essential to block out any distractions, such as other conversations nearby, and avoid checking your phone, as these actions can detract from active listening. Also, try not to immediately impose your ideas or solutions as the patient is telling you their story. Instead, allow them the space to fully express themselves without interruption or premature judgment. By refraining from jumping in with your own ideas, advice, or solutions too quickly, you demonstrate respect for their perspective and show that you are genuinely interested in understanding their concerns. This relationship-centred approach fosters a more collaborative and trusting relationship, ultimately leading to better outcomes in their healthcare journey.

Active listening does involve asking relevant questions though to demonstrate understanding and clarify any uncertainties. When asking questions, it's important to wait for the speaker to pause and then inquire about specific points using open-ended questions such as "How did that make you feel?" or "What did you do next?" Open-ended questions encourage the speaker to elaborate and express themselves more freely. It's also crucial to paraphrase and summarise what has been said to confirm understanding and allow the speaker to correct any misunderstandings. When paraphrasing, it's best to start sentences with phrases like "It sounds like you're saying..." or "It seems like..." to reflect the speaker's message accurately. Additionally, I highly recommend avoiding asking *Why* questions where possible, as they may come across as accusatory and can easily incite defensiveness on the part of the patient. Instead, rephrase *Why* questions into *What* or *How* questions to promote a more collaborative and non-threatening conversation. For example, instead of asking, "Why did you do that?" you could ask, "What led you to make that decision?", "What made you decide to do that?" or "How did you come to that decision/conclusion?". If there is something the patient isn't doing, instead of asking "Why didn't you..." or "Why aren't you...? you could ask "What's holding you back from...", "What's stopping you from..." etc. While this shift in language may seem subtle, it has a powerful effect. It moves the emphasis away from the individual as the problem and instead places it on the decision or action itself, creating a degree of emotional distance that allows the patient to reflect more openly and honestly. This small but significant adjustment in language fosters a supportive and empathetic environment — one that encourages disclosure, reduces shame, and deepens the trust between clinician and patient. In practice, this might manifest as a doctor who, through keen observation and reflective questioning, discerns the stressors exacerbating a patient's chronic condition, thereby tailoring the treatment plan to address these underlying issues. This approach not only enhances the accuracy of diagnoses — by increasing the chances of uncovering the root cause of the patient's issue rather than simply treating the symptoms they're presenting with — but also reinforces the patient's sense of being seen and valued, further strengthening the therapeutic alliance.

Becoming an active listener requires deliberate practice and dedication, as old habits can be challenging to change. One effective way to cultivate this skill is by committing to summarising the key points or outcomes after each conversation or meeting for a week. This intentional effort helps solidify the habit of active listening and reinforces its importance in our interactions. With consistent practice, active listening can become a natural part of our communication style, enhancing our ability to connect with others and understand their perspectives more deeply. This in turn fosters trust and rapport but also enhances the quality of care provided, as it enables us to better understand our patients' needs and tailor treatment plans accordingly.

FEEDBACK LOOPS IN CLINICAL CONVERSATIONS

Feedback loops, essential for clarifying understanding and intentions, rely on the reciprocal exchange of information, where messages are not merely transmitted but also received, processed, and responded to. In the context of patient interactions, this might involve a healthcare professional summarising the patient's concerns to confirm accuracy, subsequently adjusting the care plan based on the patient's feedback. Similarly, within the realm of team collaborations (to be discussed further in later chapters), feedback loops ensure that all members are aligned in their understanding and approach, minimising the risk of miscommunication and errors. The efficacy of these loops hinges on the willingness to listen actively, to question constructively, and to respond thoughtfully, creating a dynamic environment where clarity and consensus are pursued with diligence.

COLLABORATIVE LISTENING IN MULTIDISCIPLINARY TEAMS

In busy multidisciplinary teams, active listening is one of the simplest but most effective tools we must build trust, foster collaboration, and deliver genuinely holistic patient care. When team members take the time to really hear one another — not just waiting for their turn to speak but truly engaging with the ideas being shared — it brings together a wealth of perspectives that no single clinician could offer alone. This kind of listening creates space for each person to contribute their unique expertise, allowing for more thoughtful and well-rounded decision-making.

For example, imagine a case conference involving a patient recovering from surgery who is also experiencing signs of depression. The surgeon might focus on the physical healing, while the nurse brings up concerns about the patient's withdrawal and low mood. The allied health team — perhaps a physiotherapist and a social worker — might mention that the patient has been hesitant to engage in rehab or has financial stressors affecting their recovery. When each of these voices is heard and acknowledged, the team is far more likely to come up with a care plan that supports the *whole* patient, not just their presenting symptoms.

It's easy to fall into a pattern where we're half-listening, especially during busy handovers or meetings where time is short. But in those moments, if we're actively tuned in, we can catch the subtle but crucial points that can change the course of a patient's care. Active listening becomes the glue that holds the team together — it fosters mutual respect, helps prevent misunderstandings, and allows for more agile and responsive care. At its core, it's about showing that each team member's perspective is not only valid but essential to delivering truly relationship-centred care.

2.4 Body Language and Non-Verbal Cues in Patient Care

"The most important thing in communication is hearing what isn't said."

— Peter F. Drucker

WHAT OUR BODIES SAY BEFORE WE SPEAK

Body language includes the full range of non-verbal cues we convey through facial expressions, posture, gestures, and eye contact. In healthcare — where emotions run high and patients often feel vulnerable — these silent signals are often more powerful than the words we speak. They can offer reassurance, demonstrate empathy, and build trust without a single sentence being uttered.

Used skilfully, body language can transform a routine clinical interaction into one of comfort and connection. But when we're unaware of our own non-verbal cues — or fail to read and respond to those of our patients — we risk creating distance or misunderstanding. As communication expert James Borg famously noted, while the exact statistics are debated, the majority of our communication comes not from what we say, but how we say it — including tone, facial expression, and body language.

Mastering this unspoken language isn't just a nice-to-have — it's a critical part of emotionally intelligent, relationship-centred care.

READING THE UNSPOKEN: DETECTING AND INTERPRETING PATIENT BODY LANGUAGE

To truly connect with our patients, we need to listen with more than just our ears. The ability to detect and interpret body language allows us to tune in to emotions that may never be verbally expressed — but which are no less important to address. These subtle, non-verbal cues often reveal fear, pain, anxiety, or emotional distress, giving us insight into a patient's inner experience even before they speak a word.

Fidgeting or restless movements might signal unease. Avoiding eye contact could reflect shame, guilt, or discomfort. A clenched jaw or rigid posture may point to pain or apprehension. These cues aren't always obvious, but with practice and intentional awareness, we can become more adept at spotting them and responding with empathy and care.

Developing this skill takes time and reflection. Role-playing, observation exercises, and feedback sessions — whether formal or informal — can sharpen our ability to "read the room." Just as important is the mindset we bring, curiosity over assumption, and patience over judgment. Our goal isn't to diagnose emotions at a glance, but to notice when something feels off and create space for the patient to express what they may not yet know how to say.

These moments show up everywhere. In the hospital, a patient turning away or folding their arms may be bracing for bad news. In a GP clinic, someone slouched and silent might be carrying emotional weight that has nothing to do with their symptoms. In mental health settings, even a slight flicker in facial expression can indicate a shift in mood or openness.

When we become fluent in this unspoken language, our care becomes more attuned — not just to the body, but to the whole person. It's a skill that strengthens trust, deepens connection, and ultimately leads to better outcomes for both the patient and the practitioner.

MIRRORING TO BUILD CONNECTION

Earlier, we touched on the mirror neuron system — a network in the brain that activates both when we perform an action and when we observe someone else doing the same — which plays a crucial role in empathy and social connection. This system forms the neurological basis for a powerful communication technique: mirroring.

Mirroring is a natural, often subconscious behaviour in which we reflect the gestures, posture, tone, or facial expressions of the person we're interacting with. Humans tend to do this instinctively when we feel connected or in sync with someone. This unconscious mimicry helps build trust and rapport because, on a biological level, we tend to feel safer and more at ease with those who seem similar to us. Conversely, we're often more guarded around those who appear very different. Mirroring leverages this principle by creating a subtle sense of alignment.

When used intentionally in healthcare, mirroring becomes a gentle but powerful way to show empathy and attentiveness. For instance, if a patient leans forward to speak more earnestly, subtly reflecting that posture — without exaggeration — can reinforce that you're present and engaged. Matching their tone of voice, pace of speech, or emotional energy can also help them feel seen and understood.

But mirroring can be more than a passive, empathetic response — it can also be used strategically to build and test for rapport. This involves what's known in communication theory as pacing and leading. Initially, you "pace" the interaction by matching the patient's posture, energy, or tone. Once a sense of connection is established, you gently shift your own body language — perhaps by leaning back or adjusting your posture — and observe whether the patient follows your lead. If they mirror you within twenty to thirty seconds, it's often a sign that rapport has been built.

Of course, this art requires a delicate balance. Over-exaggerated or insincere mirroring can feel disingenuous, even manipulative. The key lies in subtlety and authentic presence — aiming not to copy, but to resonate with the patient's emotional state. When done well, mirroring becomes a quiet yet powerful language of connection — one that fosters mutual understanding, emotional safety, and trust.

THE BRIDGE TO CONNECTION

To help healthcare professionals integrate the practice of mirroring into patient care, the mnemonic BRIDGE offers a helpful guide. Each letter represents a key dimension of non-verbal connection that, when used intentionally, can strengthen rapport and build trust.

B – Body Posture

Subtly mirroring a patient's posture can create a sense of alignment and mutual understanding. If a patient is sitting with their arms crossed, briefly matching this stance before gently uncrossing your own arms can signal empathy and encourage openness — without needing to say a word.

R – Rhythm (Speech Pacing)

Pacing your speech to match the patient's rhythm can help put them at ease. Slowing down with an anxious patient can create calm, while mirroring a livelier rhythm with an upbeat patient can build energy and rapport. It's not about mimicking — it's about meeting the patient where they are.

I – Interactions (Touch)

Appropriate and respectful touch — such as a light hand on the shoulder or arm — can powerfully mirror emotional tone. When used thoughtfully, this form of connection can convey warmth, reassurance, and presence, especially in emotionally charged situations.

D – Demeanour (Facial Expression, Tone, Language)

Our facial expressions, tone of voice, and even word choice deeply impact how patients interpret our intentions. The face offers a wealth of non-verbal information; even the slightest movements can convey approval, disapproval, happiness, anger, fear, or disgust. For instance, frowning while reading a chart — even unintentionally — can provoke anxiety, especially if the patient has just received reassuring words. The more complex the patient's medical situation, the more conscious we must be about our facial expressions.

Reflecting a patient's demeanour encompasses more than just facial expressions — it also involves mirroring their tone of voice and language. If a patient speaks softly and slowly, doing the same in return communicates empathy and attentiveness. Using language that echoes the patient's own phrasing when discussing symptoms or treatment options can enhance rapport. Conversely, adapting a concerned tone or validating their worries with appropriate language can help the patient feel heard and supported.

G – Gestures

"Your brain is 12.5 times more likely to believe my gesture over my words," says body language expert Vanessa Van Edwards. Gestures such as nodding, mirroring hand movements, or using similar physical cues during conversation can subconsciously affirm the bond between provider and patient. These subtle actions reinforce the message that you are truly present.

E – Energy (Emotional Mirroring)

Perhaps the most powerful element of all is emotional mirroring — genuinely sharing in a patient's excitement, frustration, or grief. When a patient feels that their emotions are not only understood but reflected, trust deepens. Acknowledging their joy, fear, or disappointment strengthens the human connection at the heart of healing.

By intentionally applying the BRIDGE framework, we create a richer, more empathetic connection with our patients. And it's not just about matching their state — it's also about gently leading them toward calm and reassurance. Mirroring, when done thoughtfully, can work both ways.

Just as we can reflect our patients' body language, tone, and energy, we can also influence theirs. By projecting calm through our own posture, gestures, and tone, we activate the patient's mirror neuron system in a way that promotes relaxation and emotional regulation.

I remember a patient who returned after a root canal procedure that, unfortunately, hadn't resolved her pain. She arrived upset, accompanied by her equally frustrated husband. Their body language was tense, their tone sharp. Rather than react defensively, I grounded myself in calm. I acknowledged their frustration and mirrored their emotional state with sincere empathy — soft tone, steady posture, open gestures. Gradually, the tension began to dissipate. They softened. We were able to have a constructive, respectful conversation and explore the next steps in her treatment plan together. That moment was a testament to the quiet power of emotional mirroring — not just to de-escalate conflict, but to transform it into collaboration.

BODY LANGUAGE DO'S AND DON'TS

When it comes to using body language to build trust and connection, a few simple principles can make a profound difference. Paying attention to how we present ourselves physically — our posture, eye contact, gestures, and proximity — can either open the door to genuine connection or unintentionally create distance. It's worth being mindful of these small but powerful cues, especially in healthcare, where our non-verbal communication often speaks louder than our words.

Among the do's, maintaining open body posture stands paramount, inviting dialogue and signalling receptiveness. Nods and smiles, when genuine, affirm understanding and empathy, reinforcing the patient's sense of being valued and heard. Importantly, smiles need to be authentic — the kind that reaches the eyes — because patients can instinctively detect when warmth is forced or superficial.

Leaning forward slightly during a conversation conveys attentiveness and shows you're engaged, without being overly intense. Similarly, a head tilt — often overlooked — can be a powerful sign of curiosity and empathy. Research even suggests that delivering bad news with a head tilt makes you appear more likable and compassionate, helping the patient better receive difficult information.

Proximity also plays a key role in non-verbal communication. A comfortable distance is typically about an arm's length apart — close enough to shake hands if needed, but far enough to respect personal space. Standing too close can feel intrusive or overly intimate, especially when a patient is already feeling vulnerable.

Eye contact, when used judiciously, communicates engagement and sincerity, though it should be modulated to respect cultural norms and individual comfort. A steady gaze can convey attentiveness, while intermittent glances away can prevent the interaction from feeling too intense or invasive.

In addition to managing eye contact, we can enhance our ability to focus fully on our patients by leveraging supportive tools. For instance, utilising a team member — like a dental assistant — to take notes during consultations allows us to be fully present. For those without support staff, technologies like Heidi Health or other similar tools can streamline administrative tasks. Heidi Health's AI-powered tools, such as Heidi Scribe, automate the transcription of consultations into clinical notes and action items. This frees clinicians to maintain uninterrupted eye contact and promotes active listening, ensuring patients receive undivided attention and fostering a deeper connection built on trust and empathy. It has been a game-changer in my clinical practice. As healthcare evolves, I truly believe that embracing and integrating such technologies not only enhances efficiency by reducing the time spent on administration and other activities unrelated to patient care but also enriches the quality of our patient-provider interactions, ultimately improving healthcare delivery.

Among the don'ts, avoid gestures that may be perceived as dismissive, dominant, or disconnected — such as pointing, crossing your arms, checking your watch, or standing over a seated patient. These can unintentionally signal impatience, disinterest, or a power imbalance. Similarly, excessive device usage during consultations — like typing notes into a computer while a patient is speaking — can create barriers that undermine rapport. It gives the impression that the patient isn't your primary focus, potentially causing them to withhold information or feel unheard. We must remain vigilant to our body language and continuously refine our non-verbal communication skills to ensure we foster, rather than hinder, meaningful connections with our patients.

When I was a newly graduated associate dentist, I spent one day a week shadowing a senior dentist at the group practice where I worked. During one new patient exam, I observed him sitting parallel to the patient with his arms crossed, legs stretched out, chin in hand, and gaze fixed down at the wall. He nodded occasionally, barely speaking except for the odd "mmm" sound. I remember feeling awkward just watching — so I can only imagine how the patient felt. His lack of engagement and closed-off posture likely left the patient feeling disregarded and wondering if she was even being heard.

Personally, I've chosen to adopt a different approach. I position myself diagonally opposite the patient, maintaining eye contact and showing that I am fully engaged in their care. Over time, I've learned to memorise key aspects of our conversations, or alternatively, I utilise the help of my dental assistant or technology like Heidi Health to take notes, so I can give my full attention to the person in front of me. I've also noticed how common it is for clinicians — particularly GPs — to speak to patients while focused on their screen. While often necessary, this habit creates both a physical and emotional barrier to building trust and rapport, as it can make patients feel secondary or ignored during their consultation. Further, without being fully engaged with our patients, we may miss subtle signs in their body language that could reveal how they're feeling or that they might be holding something back. This means we risk losing the patient's trust or missing their full story altogether. We can't provide the right level of care to our patients if they do not feel comfortable enough to tell us everything, so it is imperative that we create a safe space for them to do so.

In dentistry, I often see another common disconnect: clinicians explaining procedures or diagnoses to patients who are lying in the dental chair — sometimes fully supine, other times semi-reclined —

while the dentist stands over them, sits beside them, or even speaks to them from behind. Now imagine yourself in the patient's shoes — lying back in a chair, possibly feeling anxious or vulnerable, while someone stands over you or speaks from behind. It's not exactly the ideal setup for open, two way communication, is it? Whether the provider is speaking from beside them or standing behind, this disempowers the patient and limits their ability to engage. This approach can significantly impact the patient's experience and their ability to absorb the information being relayed effectively because this positioning can make the patient feel vulnerable and exposed, both physically and psychologically. They may find it challenging to maintain eye contact or even see the dentist's facial expressions, which are crucial for understanding empathy and reassurance. Moreover, having the dentist speak from behind rather than facing the patient directly further exacerbates the disconnect. Communication is hindered as the patient may struggle to hear clearly or follow the details of the explanation. This setup can lead to feelings of discomfort, unease, and even distrust, as it creates a perception that the dentist is not fully engaging with them or prioritising their understanding making it less likely the patient will feel comfortable proceeding with the proposed treatment.

It's easy to forget that patients may arrive burdened by overwhelm, anxiety, fear, or other difficult emotions in many healthcare environments. The above-mentioned seemingly minor aspects of interaction do have a profound psychological impact on our patients, especially in environments where the patient is already feeling psychologically and physically vulnerable such as the dental setting. They contribute to the overall atmosphere of the dental visit and shape the patient's perception of the clinician's empathy and professionalism. To foster a strong relationship between clinician and patient, we need to consider these nuances in communication and physical positioning. By being more intentional with how we carry ourselves, we foster stronger therapeutic alliances that benefit both patient and provider. At the end of the day, patients may not remember every word we say — but they'll always remember how we made them feel.

And often, that feeling starts with how we show up before we even speak.

2.5 Emotional Awareness in Diagnosis and Treatment Planning

"When awareness is brought to an emotion, power is brought to your life."

— Tara Meyer Robson

In healthcare, it's easy to focus on what's measurable — vital signs, lab results, physical symptoms. But beneath the surface, our patients' emotional and psychological states often hold equally important clues to their overall well-being.

The importance of recognising emotional expressions as windows into underlying health issues cannot be overstated as it helps us understand our patients more completely and holistically. A furrowed brow or averted gaze may speak volumes about a patient's discomfort or fear. These subtle cues, when noticed and interpreted with empathy, offer insight that deepens our understanding of the patient's experience. This emotional data, often overlooked in a purely symptom-focused approach, can reveal connections between mental stress and physical symptoms that might otherwise go unnoticed. For instance, the manifestation of irritable bowel syndrome (IBS) can often be entwined with anxiety or depression, conditions that might not be immediately apparent without a keen sensitivity to the patient's emotional cues.

In practice, many of these cues are easy to miss, especially in time-pressured environments. Yet they can offer vital insight into how a patient is really feeling. For example, you might notice:

- Hesitation before answering a question
- A forced smile or overly polite responses
- Sudden changes in voice tone, energy, or posture
- Nervous laughter or avoiding eye contact after difficult topics
- Fidgeting, sighing, or other signs of internal tension

These seemingly minor behaviours can be signs of anxiety, discomfort, fear, or even unspoken concerns. When we take a moment to tune in, we're better equipped to respond with empathy — and ask the right follow-up questions that can help patients open up and feel understood.

Integrating emotional intelligence into diagnosis allows us to take a truly holistic approach — recognising each patient as a whole person made up of body, mind, and spirit. This comprehensive perspective not only enriches the understanding of the patient's condition but also enhances the therapeutic relationship. When our patients feel that their emotional and psychological states are acknowledged and valued, they are more likely to engage openly and honestly in the diagnostic process, providing us with a fuller picture of their health.

Moreover, incorporating emotional intelligence into diagnosis facilitates a more compassionate approach to patient care. It enables us to tailor our communication and intervention strategies to the individual needs and emotional states of our patients, thereby optimising the care experience. For example, a patient grappling with a new diagnosis of diabetes may experience a range of emotions, from denial to despair. An emotionally intelligent approach to care recognises these emotions, addressing them with sensitivity and providing support that encompasses both the management of the disease and the emotional resilience of the patient.

This empathetic engagement extends beyond the individual patient, reaching out to embrace the family and wider support network. For example, when a child comes in for a routine dental check-up, the parents might believe everything is fine, only to learn that the child has multiple cavities and requires treatment under general anaesthetic by a specialist. This news can be shocking and deeply concerning for the parents. In these moments, emotional intelligence becomes critical — not just in managing the child's needs, but in recognising the emotional weight the parents are likely carrying. Many parents feel a deep sense of guilt or failure upon hearing news like this — even when there was nothing they could have done to prevent it. That's why it's so important to approach these conversations without judgement. Creating a safe, supportive space allows parents to ask questions, express their concerns, and feel reassured that the focus is on solutions — not blame. By responding with empathy, clear communication, and genuine care, we can build trust and foster an environment of mutual respect and collaboration. In doing so, the treatment process transforms into a shared journey, where everyone is working together toward the common goal of the child's health and well-being.

The benefits of this emotionally intelligent approach to diagnosis are manifold. It not only improves the accuracy of diagnoses by considering the full spectrum of the patient's experience but also enhances patient compliance and satisfaction. Patients who feel understood and supported are more likely to adhere to treatment plans and engage in positive health behaviours, leading to better outcomes. This approach therefore promotes a more fulfilling professional experience for us as healthcare professionals, as we can find deeper meaning and satisfaction in our work when we can connect with our patients on an emotional level.

In practice, the development of emotional intelligence skills requires both education and reflection. Consider training programs that emphasise the importance of empathy, active listening, and emotional self-awareness which can equip us as practitioners with the tools we need to incorporate emotional insights into our diagnostic approach. Additionally, reflective practice, in which we regularly assess our interactions with patients and our own emotional responses, can foster a greater sensitivity to the emotional dimensions of patient care. We will discuss this in detail in later chapters.

As healthcare technology evolves, especially with the rise of artificial intelligence (AI), emotional intelligence becomes more essential — not less. While machines can assist in analysing symptoms and data, they cannot replicate the warmth, intuition, and human connection required for truly compassionate care. The ability to see beyond symptoms, to connect with patients emotionally, and to consider their psychological state is not a bonus feature of good care — it is its very foundation.

2.6 Navigating Difficult Conversations with Compassion

> *"When dealing with people, remember you are not dealing with creatures of logic, but with creatures of emotion."*
>
> — Dale Carnegie

Navigating difficult conversations with patients and families requires far more than clinical expertise — it demands emotional intelligence, empathy, and an unwavering commitment to human connection. It's about reading the room — sensing the fear behind a stoic facade, the flicker of hope behind anxious eyes, or the silence that speaks louder than words. It's about responding not just with facts, but with sensitivity, compassion, and an understanding of the emotional journey that patients and their families are navigating.

At the heart of these conversations lies empathy — the ability not just to understand, but to genuinely *feel* with patients. True empathy requires active listening: hearing not only the words spoken but the emotions underneath. It's about fostering a mentality that we are all on the same team, standing alongside patients rather than speaking at them.

PREPARING FOR DIFFICULT CONVERSATIONS

Effective communication during emotionally charged moments begins well before the conversation itself. Preparation involves reflecting not only on the patient's medical history and clinical facts but also on their emotional journey to this point. What's their current understanding of their condition? What emotional supports do they have — or lack? How do they typically respond to stress or change? Anticipating potential questions, concerns, and emotional reactions allows us to craft a communication strategy that is both informative and compassionate.

A quick tip when preparing for a difficult conversation: jot down three things — what the patient needs to know, what they might be feeling, and how you'll support them emotionally.

Equally important is checking in with your own emotional state before entering the conversation. Patients can sense tension, defensiveness, or discomfort — so grounding yourself first can make a big difference.

TIMING, PACING, AND EMOTIONAL AWARENESS

Mastering the art of timing and pacing is crucial. For example, when seeing a new patient who has been with their previous dentist for years and believes that everything is fine, it can be challenging to find undiagnosed issues like gum disease or failing fillings. It's important not to judge the patient or their previous dentist, as this will likely reflect poorly on you as the new provider. Instead, gently bring up the findings, using x-rays, photos, or scans to show the patient what you're seeing without overwhelming them or pushing for a lot of treatment right away. It might be more effective to plant the seed of these issues and build trust over time. As long as it's clinically safe, you can revisit the concerns at a future visit once you've had the chance to build rapport, the patient feels more comfortable and has had time to process the information. By pacing these conversations thoughtfully, we can avoid overwhelming patients and allow them the time to absorb, reflect, and ask questions without feeling rushed or ambushed. Silence and pauses should not be feared — they are often the spaces where understanding begins to take root.

LANGUAGE AND FRAMING MATTER

When delivering unfavourable news or discussing complex treatment options, the words we choose matter immensely. Our language should be simple and clear, yet compassionate — avoiding jargon that could alienate or overwhelm, while still respecting the seriousness of the situation. In doing so, we honour both the patient's intelligence and their emotional state.

Rather than dictating a course of action, it's important to use language that invites collaboration — for example, "What we're seeing suggests that..." or "One option we could consider is...". Compare:

- "You have severe gum disease, and we need to act fast."

vs.

- "Your gums are showing signs of infection, and we have a few options we can explore together to get them healthy again."

These subtle shifts move the conversation from a one-sided delivery of information to a shared decision-making process. They reframe the dynamic from expert vs. patient to a therapeutic partnership. Patients feel more respected, more involved, and more empowered to take an active role in their care.

THE POWER OF ACTIVE, GENUINE LISTENING AND EMPATHETIC RESPONSES

As we've explored, the foundation of compassionate communication is listening to understand — not just waiting to respond. This shift transforms interactions from transactional exchanges to meaningful human connections.

A few simple techniques can help: pausing before replying to fully absorb what the patient said, summarising key points to confirm your understanding, and using open-ended questions that invite dialogue. Instead of asking, "Do you have any questions?" — which often leads to a reflexive "no" — try, "What questions do you have?" This subtle change encourages patients to speak up and engage more deeply in their care.

I once worked with an associate dentist who, on the surface, seemed bubbly and kind — always smiling and friendly. Yet after returning from maternity leave, I began receiving unexpected negative feedback from her patients. When I asked my assistant for her insight, she mentioned that the dentist didn't come across as genuine. Patients could sense the disconnect and lack of sincerity, and many left feeling unsettled. It was a powerful reminder that people can feel when we're putting on a façade — and true empathy can't be faked. No matter how well we phrase our words, if our presence isn't sincere, patients will feel it — and without trust, no technique or script can bridge that gap.

Crafting empathetic responses isn't about finding the perfect words — it's about being fully present. A thoughtful reply might begin by acknowledging the patient's emotional state — "It's completely understandable to feel anxious about this procedure..." — followed by addressing the concern — "Here's how we make it as comfortable as possible..." — and concluding with an invitation to continue the conversation. This structure not only reassures the patient but empowers them through understanding. It also gives us an opportunity to correct any misconceptions and ensure our message has truly landed.

The words we use can either build connection or unintentionally create distance and undermine trust. Here are some common phrases to be mindful of — and their more empathetic alternatives:

DON'TS **Avoid Saying**	DO'S **Try Saying Instead**
"Do you have any questions?"	"What questions do you have?"
"You need to..."	"One option we could consider is..."
"There's nothing to worry about."	"It's completely understandable to feel concerned. Let's talk about it."
"It's standard procedure."	"Here's what to expect and how we'll support you through it."
"You should have come in sooner."	"I'm glad you came in today — let's focus on next steps together."
"It's not a big deal."	"I understand this might feel overwhelming. I'm here to guide you."

By creating a space where the patient feels safe to ask questions, we enhance their sense of control and partnership in the decision-making process. When patients feel heard, understood, and included, they're far more likely to engage in their care, voice their concerns, and make informed choices. That's the power of listening — not as a communication tactic, but as a genuine act of human connection.

NON-VERBAL COMMUNICATION: THE UNSPOKEN MESSAGE

As discussed earlier, body language and tone of voice are powerful tools in building connection — but they become especially critical during emotionally charged or difficult conversations. In these moments, even subtle cues can have a significant impact on how a message is received.

Sitting at the same level as the patient — rather than towering over them — helps create a sense of equality and safety. Maintaining warm, steady eye contact (without being overbearing), using a calm, reassuring tone, and speaking at a measured pace can help anxious patients stay grounded. Conversely, a rushed tone, crossed arms, or frequently glancing at your watch can unintentionally signal impatience or detachment — even when that's not your intent.

When our non-verbal cues align with our verbal messages, we communicate compassion, confidence, and care — often without saying a word.

BUILDING TRUST THROUGH COMPASSIONATE DIALOGUE

Trust isn't built overnight — it's built interaction by interaction, word by word. Every time we approach a difficult conversation with sensitivity, transparency, and respect, we strengthen that foundation.

It's crucial that patients understand they are not passive recipients of care but active participants in their health journey, which can significantly ease the burden of making tough decisions. Engaging them collaboratively promotes a sense of control and empowerment, even in situations where the news may not be ideal. It is important to always acknowledge their emotions first before diving into facts. Then, by presenting all available options clearly and fairly, discussing potential outcomes, and respecting the patient's values and preferences, we empower them to take an active role in their care. This approach not only enhances their sense of control and autonomy but also fosters a deeper trust in the healthcare team. It's important to remember that our role is not to decide what's right for the patient, but to provide clear information, outline the pros and cons, and support them in making their own decisions. We need to respect their autonomy, even when patients choose a path different from what we might recommend. That said, professionalism must remain intact: we are not obligated to provide treatment that we believe is inappropriate, unsafe, or beyond our expertise — even if a patient insists. In those cases, it's important to respectfully decline and offer appropriate referrals, preserving both patient safety and professional integrity. These conversations require sensitivity, as they touch on the delicate balance between patient autonomy and professional responsibility. We must also commit to being honest about what we know and don't know and committing to finding answers where needed.

When patients feel genuinely heard, respected, and cared for, they are more likely to engage meaningfully in their treatment, share important information, and trust the process — even when the road is difficult.

CASE STUDIES IN COMPASSIONATE CONVERSATIONS

The power of empathy in addressing patient concerns is perhaps best illustrated through case studies that reflect real-world scenarios. One such case involves James, a 52-year-old man who was recently diagnosed with type 2 diabetes. Initially, James was in denial, feeling overwhelmed and fearful about how this diagnosis would impact his daily life, especially his ability to enjoy family gatherings and his love for cooking. Recognising the emotional turmoil he was experiencing, the healthcare team employed active listening and empathetic communication to delve into his concerns. They acknowledged James's fear of needing to give up his favourite foods and the potential impact on his relationships with family members who enjoyed dining out together. Through a series of supportive conversations that combined empathy with education about disease management — such as incorporating healthier versions of his favourite dishes — the team helped James gradually move toward acceptance and active participation in his care plan. They even worked with him to develop meal plans that included nutritious alternatives, allowing him to enjoy cooking without sacrificing his health.

Another case highlights the role of empathy in cross-cultural care, involving Aisha, a 30-year-old woman from a Muslim background who was hesitant to discuss her reproductive health issues. Aisha held cultural beliefs that made her reluctant to seek help for what she perceived as a personal and private matter. Aisha's doctor, aware of these cultural nuances, took the time to engage Aisha in a dialogue aimed at understanding her concerns within the context of her beliefs. They approached the conversation with sensitivity, assuring Aisha that her values were respected and emphasising that seeking help was a sign of strength, not weakness. This respectful approach facilitated a deeper connection, allowing Aisha to express her fears about stigmatisation and the impact of her condition on her future family planning. As a result, her doctor was able to tailor the care plan to align with Aisha's values, which enhanced her engagement and compliance with the treatment recommendations.

These cases underscore the transformative potential of empathy in healthcare, demonstrating how sensitive and empathetic communication can navigate the complexities of patient concerns. By fostering an environment where trust, understanding, and collaboration thrive, we can pave the way to healing. Addressing patient concerns with this level of depth and care not only affirms our commitment to the physical well-being of those we serve but also acknowledges the emotional and psychological dimensions of health that are equally vital to recovery and overall well-being.

2.7 Enhancing Patient Compliance Through Trust and Empathy

> *"The only way to change someone's mind is to connect with them from the heart."*
>
> — Rasheed Ogunlaru

UNDERSTANDING PATIENT PERSPECTIVES

At the heart of enhancing patient compliance is the need to truly understand each patient's unique perspective, a goal that calls for genuine curiosity and emotional intelligence. Patients bring with them a lifetime of experiences, beliefs, and — sometimes — deep-seated fears that can shape their approach to healthcare. By tapping into these narratives and connecting on a human level, we can uncover the emotional roots that influence their choices, allowing us to tailor our communication and recommendations in ways that resonate deeply and ultimately increase their willingness to engage in their care.

For instance, I had a patient who was adamant about not having a crown placed due to a bad experience in the past. She was convinced that a crown would lead to losing her tooth and felt that extraction was the only option. Rather than pushing back directly, I tapped into emotional intelligence, listening carefully and acknowledging her concerns. Through open conversation and empathy, I reassured her about the procedure, addressing her past fears. Ultimately, she trusted me enough to go forward with the crown — and now, she jokingly calls it the "queen of her mouth," her favourite tooth of all. It wasn't about me wanting to save the tooth more than she did, or about convincing her to choose what I thought was the best treatment option. It was about creating space for her to make a decision based on understanding, not fear. If she had still wanted to have the tooth removed after that conversation, I absolutely would have supported that. The goal was never to push — it was to ensure she felt informed, heard, and in control of her own care.

MOTIVATIONAL INTERVIEWING WITH AN EQ APPROACH

Motivational interviewing is one of the most effective techniques we can use to enhance patient compliance. It's more than a method; it's a mindset, built on principles of emotional intelligence that help patients identify and articulate their own reasons for sticking with treatment plans. Through carefully guided questions and reflective listening, motivational interviewing allows patients to explore their ambivalence, voice their concerns, and eventually identify their own motivation for change. For example, rather than telling a patient why a treatment is important, we might ask them how their condition impacts their daily life or what their health goals are. You might also ask them to explain in their own words what going ahead with or delaying treatment could mean for them. This technique respects their autonomy and fosters a collaborative, empathetic dialogue. It gently helps patients resolve ambivalence and take ownership of their care. It also creates a therapeutic alliance where the patient feels genuinely heard and understood, paving the way for better adherence to recommendations and greater satisfaction with their care.

BUILDING A COLLABORATIVE CARE PLAN

Recognising patients as the experts of their own experiences, we invite them to co-create a realistic and personalised care plan that reflects their values and preferences. This kind of collaboration ensures the plan aligns with what matters most to them and addresses any concerns that might otherwise become barriers to compliance. By thoughtfully listening to their input and weaving their goals into the process, we foster a shared sense of responsibility that strengthens their commitment to follow through. When patients help shape their care plan, they're not just more likely to stick with it — they're more likely to feel seen, respected, and empowered.

EMPATHETIC ENGAGEMENT WITH PATIENTS AND FAMILIES

This approach recognises the family as integral to the patient's journey, experiencing their own spectrum of emotions — fear, hope, despair. Engaging empathetically with families involves acknowledging their concerns, offering comfort, and, crucially, involving them in care discussions. Such inclusion not only bolsters the patient's support system but also demystifies the healthcare process, building a foundation of trust and cooperation.

This is especially true in dentistry, where families often play a vital role in supporting children, elderly patients, or those with special needs. By acknowledging the concerns and emotions of family members, dentists can create a supportive environment that eases anxiety and fosters cooperation during dental visits. Involving families in discussions about treatment plans, oral hygiene routines, and preventive care measures not only empowers them to contribute to the patient's oral health but also strengthens the bond of trust between the dental team and the entire family unit. This inclusive approach ensures that patients receive comprehensive support, both inside and outside the dental office, ultimately leading to improved oral health outcomes. When families feel included and respected, it strengthens the bond between the practice and the people we serve.

ADDRESSING COMPLIANCE CHALLENGES WITH EMPATHY

Even with the best intentions, compliance challenges often arise, and it's here that emotional intelligence becomes crucial. Addressing these challenges with empathy means truly understanding the barriers each patient faces — whether they're logistical, emotional, or due to a lack of information. Avoid making assumptions about why a patient is non-compliant. Instead, ask open-ended questions to uncover the root cause — only then can we work together to find an appropriate solution. By approaching these situations with an open heart and mind, we can help our patients problem-solve in ways that feel supportive rather than directive. For instance, if a patient struggles to keep appointments due to a busy schedule, we might work together to find a more convenient time or arrange follow-up calls to keep them engaged in their care. This kind of empathetic problem-solving not only tackles immediate barriers but also reinforces their trust in us, which is key to fostering long-term commitment to their health journey.

For example, I currently have a patient with autism undergoing clear aligner treatment and was adamant against fixed braces. Compliance is essential to the success of clear aligner orthodontic treatment, yet he's struggled with various challenges throughout the process. Rather than getting frustrated at the slow rate of progress with treatment, we've worked together on strategies to make the treatment more manageable, such as longer wear times (14 days instead of 7) and scheduling more frequent appointments. His mother has regularly expressed her gratitude for our collaborative approach and my commitment to finding solutions, which, rather than derailing the process, has helped us keep steady progress. When we lead with empathy, curiosity, and respect for our patients' lived experiences, we build the trust that makes true healing — and real compliance — possible.

2.8 Relationship-Centred Care and The Role of EQ

"In the last decade or so, science has discovered a tremendous amount about the role emotions play in our lives. Researchers have found that even more than IQ, your emotional awareness and abilities to handle feelings will determine our success and happiness in all walks of life, including family relationships."

— John Gottman

If emotional intelligence helps us navigate individual interactions, relationship-centred care (RCC) reminds us of the broader web of connections that shape every moment in healthcare. We're all familiar with the concept of patient-centred care — an approach that emphasises respect for patient values, preferences, and involvement in decision-making. But as you've likely seen throughout this book, many of the most impactful moments in care are not just about the patient in isolation — they're about relationships. Whether it's the connection between patient and provider, between team members, or even the relationship we have with ourselves, these interactions shape the quality and depth of care we provide.

Relationship-centred care builds on the foundation of patient-centred care and takes it further, recognising that all aspects of healing are rooted in meaningful relationships — relationships between patient and clinician, among colleagues, within the broader community, and even within the clinician's relationship to self. It asks us to move beyond seeing care as a series of individual transactions and instead view it as a dynamic, interconnected process. This shift requires us as healthcare providers to be not only clinically proficient but emotionally and relationally attuned — creating environments where respect, collaboration, and compassion elevate every patient's journey through the healthcare system.

The principles of RCC outlined by Mary Catherine Beach and Thomas Inui align well with the foundational elements of patient-centred care — respect for patient values, coordination of care, communication, comfort, and access. However, RCC takes these concepts further, with four distinct principles that shape a new approach to care.

PRINCIPLE 1: RELATIONSHIPS EMBRACE PERSONHOOD BEYOND ROLES

In RCC, both the patient and clinician are seen as whole individuals, each bringing unique experiences, values, and perspectives to the care encounter. This approach calls for the clinician to be mindful of their own emotions, biases, and reactions, fostering authentic interactions grounded in genuine respect. It's not enough to merely act respectfully — RCC calls us to cultivate authentic, internal respect for every person we serve. Emotional intelligence is essential here, allowing us to perceive and respond to the deeper, often unspoken, values guiding a patient's decisions and to honour those values in every part of the care plan.

PRINCIPLE 2: AFFECT AND EMOTION AS CENTRAL COMPONENTS

RCC acknowledges that empathy and emotional support are vital in healthcare relationships, challenging the traditional notion of "detached concern." Emotional intelligence becomes a powerful tool, enabling us to connect authentically, thereby supporting patients' emotional well-being and building trust. By empathising with our patients, we can help them process their emotions, offering validation and support that can be transformative, even therapeutic, in their overall experience. This practice underscores the power of emotional presence, transforming clinical care into a deeply human, relational process.

PRINCIPLE 3: RECIPROCAL INFLUENCE IN HEALTH INTERACTIONS

Unlike isolated transactions, healthcare interactions are dynamic exchanges where each interaction influences both patient and clinician. RCC recognises that clinicians, too, grow through their relationships with patients, often gaining insights that enrich their professional and personal lives. This approach encourages us to learn from the patient, honouring their experience and fostering a mutually beneficial exchange. Emotional intelligence again plays a critical role, guiding us to remain open, flexible, and responsive, creating a balanced partnership that goes beyond a simple hierarchy of "expert" and "patient."

PRINCIPLE 4: THE MORAL FOUNDATION OF RELATIONSHIPS

RCC rests on the principle that genuine relationships are morally valuable, forming a basis for deep commitment to the well-being of others. Unlike the transactional approach of customer service, genuine relationships foster a personal investment that renews clinicians and strengthens their commitment to service. RCC urges us to go beyond mere role performance, embracing honest, genuine relationships that allow patients to sense their impact on us — not just as recipients of care, but as fellow human beings on a shared journey. Here, emotional intelligence is essential for maintaining moral integrity and authenticity in these relationships, reinforcing a deeper, morally grounded connection to each patient's care.

Just as emotional intelligence allows us to connect more deeply with individuals, relationship-centred care challenges us to see the larger tapestry of human connection that defines healthcare. By recognising the interdependence of every relationship — patient, team, community, and self — we move beyond isolated interactions toward a culture of healing, one grounded in empathy, authenticity, and mutual respect. In doing so, we don't just care for our patients more effectively; we create space for everyone in the system, ourselves included, to thrive. And perhaps most importantly, relationship-centred care reminds us that the way we relate to ourselves — through inner dialogue, self-compassion, and emotional regulation — directly affects the care we're able to offer others.

2.9 Why Empathy Improves Outcomes – for Patients, Teams, and Clinicians

---

> *"When you listen with empathy to another person, you give that person psychological air."*
>
> — Stephen R. Covey

When we take the time to truly recognise — and resonate with — the emotional states of others, something shifts. Empathy becomes more than just a skill; it becomes a guiding principle, a compass for navigating the complexities of care with compassion and sensitivity. In the complex world of healthcare, there's a crucial truth that often gets overlooked: empathy plays a vital role in the healing process. It's not just a nice-to-have or an extra layer on top of medical expertise — it's a powerful force that can significantly influence a patient's recovery. And this isn't just based on personal stories. A growing body of research shows a clear link between empathetic care and improved patient outcomes.

Research continues to reinforce what many of us witness every day in practice: empathy isn't just "nice" — it's clinically effective. Studies consistently show that patients treated by empathetic healthcare providers report higher satisfaction, better adherence to treatment, reduced anxiety, and even improved diagnostic outcomes. For example, a study published in the *British Journal of General Practice* found that diabetic patients cared for by physicians with high empathy scores achieved better control over their blood sugar levels, demonstrating how empathetic interactions can lead to measurable health improvements.

This link is not coincidental — it's physiological. When patients perceive genuine care and concern, their bodies respond. Stress hormones, which can exacerbate illness, decrease, while oxytocin — associated with trust, connection, and reduced anxiety — increases. This biochemical shift enhances both emotional well-being and the body's ability to heal.

But empathy's influence goes beyond biology. It creates a space where patients feel seen, heard, and valued — not as conditions, but as people navigating vulnerability. In that space, barriers like fear, shame, or confusion begin to fall away. Patients are more likely to express concerns, ask questions, and disclose relevant details — leading to clearer diagnoses, more tailored treatment plans, and ultimately, better outcomes.

The connection between empathy and treatment adherence can't be overstated. In the reality of day-to-day healthcare, getting someone to take their medication, follow advice, or make lifestyle changes isn't always easy. That's where trust makes all the difference. When patients feel understood and supported, they're far more likely to engage with their care. I've seen this time and again in my own practice. I often joke with patients about their oral hygiene habits — not to shame them, but to lighten the mood and create an honest, open space. That rapport turns a lecture into a conversation — and patients respond. They're more likely to follow through, make healthier choices, and actually come back for follow-ups. All of that leads to better results — not just in the short term, but in the long run too.

Importantly, the impact of empathy doesn't stop with patients. When empathy — and emotional intelligence more broadly — is woven into team dynamics and leadership, it transforms workplace culture. It fosters collaboration, strengthens morale, and reduces burnout. A culture of empathy elevates everyone: patients, teams, and clinicians alike. It creates a virtuous cycle — empathetic care improves outcomes, which deepens our commitment to empathy, fuelling a healthier, more sustainable system where everyone thrives.

Chapter 3

Leading from Within: Self-Awareness in Healthcare

3.1 Understanding Emotions: Building an Emotional Vocabulary

> *"There is no separation of mind and emotions; emotions, thinking, and learning are all linked."*
>
> — Eric Jensen

Before we can truly lead ourselves — or others — we need to understand the raw materials we're working with: our emotions.

Emotions signal what matters most. They're not good or bad in themselves; they simply provide information. Yet many of us were never formally taught how to name, process, or work with what we feel — especially in high-pressure fields like ours, where emotional suppression is often rewarded more than emotional awareness. But the truth is, understanding emotions is crucial — not just for supporting our patients with compassion, but for managing our own reactions under stress. Fluency in the language of emotion lays the foundation for self-awareness, empathy, and grounded leadership.

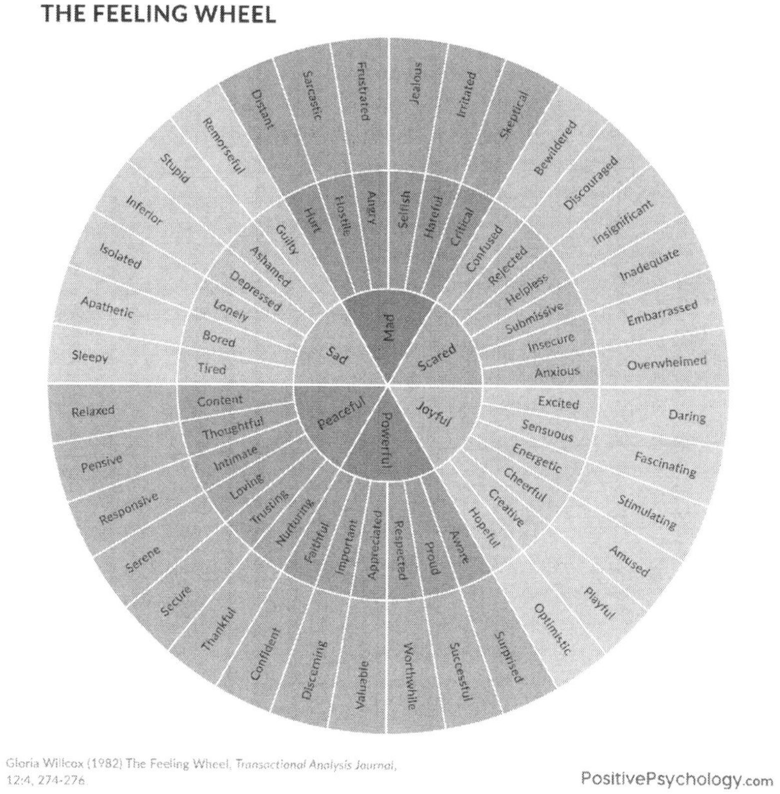

A tool that can help enormously with this is the Feeling Wheel. Originally created by Dr Gloria Willcox, the Feeling Wheel expands our emotional vocabulary beyond just "good," "bad," "happy," or "stressed." It helps us drill down into the nuances of our emotional experiences, starting with core emotions like anger, fear, joy, and sadness, and branching out into more specific feelings like frustrated, overwhelmed, hopeful, or grateful. It can be helpful to carry a hardcopy of the Feeling Wheel (see the figure below) in your diary, planner, or work bag — or simply save a digital copy to your phone. That way, you can pull it up anytime you feel an intense emotion and want to better understand it in real time.

And remember, emotions aren't neatly packaged, one-at-a-time experiences. It's completely normal to feel multiple emotions at once — even seemingly contradictory ones. You might feel hopeful *and* fearful at the same time. Or proud *and* guilty. Emotions are layered, complex, and dynamic. They're not mutually exclusive, and that's perfectly okay.

Why does this matter so much? Because being able to accurately name what we're feeling gives us power over it. Neuroscience shows that when we "name it to tame it," we engage the rational parts of our brain (like the prefrontal cortex) and dampen the reactive parts (like the amygdala). Labelling emotions literally calms the emotional centres of the brain and helps us think more clearly and respond more skilfully. It also builds self-compassion. As the saying goes, "You cannot heal what you cannot feel." When we tune into what we're really feeling, we create an opportunity to respond to ourselves with kindness. For instance, if you realise that you're feeling shame after a difficult conversation with a patient, a compassionate inner voice might say, "It's okay to feel shame. I'm a human being, and I make mistakes. This feeling is a reminder that I care, and that I can learn from this experience." Instead of ignoring or fighting the emotion, you're learning to meet it with understanding — which is the real heart of resilience.

DEEPENING YOUR UNDERSTANDING WITH AN EMOTIONAL THOUGHT TRACKER

A pre-requisite for effective, emotionally honest communication is the ability to identify our emotions and feelings. The Feeling Wheel helps us name emotions more accurately. But what if we want to go even deeper? This is where the concept of an Emotional Thought Tracker comes in.

The Emotional Thought Tracker invites us to connect emotions with the underlying thoughts that are often driving them. This personalised dictionary defines your feelings in terms of the specific thoughts that accompany and cause these feelings. Every emotion is linked to an internal story we are telling ourselves — whether we're aware of it or not.

For example:

- Anger after a clinical error might be linked to the thought: "I should never make mistakes. I'm letting everyone down."
- Anxiety before a complex procedure could come from the thought: "If I mess this up, I'll lose everyone's trust."
- Guilt when running behind schedule may be fuelled by: "I'm not doing enough. I'm failing my patients."
- Frustration with an uncooperative patient could stem from: "They should trust me by now. Why do I have to keep convincing them?"

By recognising the hidden stories behind your emotions, you have the opportunity to make sense of strong feelings instead of being swept away by them, spot unhelpful thinking patterns that can escalate emotional reactions and reframe your thoughts to create more compassion — for yourself and for others. Building your own personal Emotional Thought Tracker can be a powerful exercise in emotional self-awareness. Here's how to do it:

<u>A Practical Exercise:</u>

1. When you notice a strong emotion, pause.
2. Identify the emotion using your Feeling Wheel. If you find it difficult to put your feeling into words, try to write down

physical symptoms of your feeling, like a racing heart, shortness in breath, dullness in thinking, etc.
3. Ask: "What story am I telling myself right now that might be fuelling this feeling?"
4. Write down any thoughts listed under that feeling that you are having.
5. Reflect: Is this thought true? Is it helpful? Could I reframe it with more self-compassion or perspective?

Over time, this practice helps you catch unhelpful thoughts earlier and respond to emotional triggers with more wisdom instead of reactivity. Remember: emotions are teachers, not enemies. They aren't obstacles to being a good healthcare provider — they're essential tools for becoming an even better one.

Reflection: Deepening Your Emotional Awareness

Take a few moments to reflect on your relationship with your emotions by answering the following questions:

- *What emotions do I notice most often during my workday? Are there patterns tied to particular tasks, people, or situations?*
- *Which emotions do I tend to avoid, dismiss, or push away? Are there certain feelings that are harder for me to acknowledge?*
- *How might accurately naming my emotions help me navigate challenging moments with more calm and clarity?*
- *Have there been times when I misread my emotions — or someone else's — and how did that impact the outcome?*
- *What small step could I take this week to practice tuning into my emotions more intentionally? Maybe it's carrying a copy of the Feeling Wheel with you or simply pausing for 30 seconds during a stressful moment.*

EMOTIONAL THOUGHT TRACKER FOR HEALTHCARE PROFESSIONALS

Developing emotional intelligence starts with noticing not just what we feel, but also the thoughts and stories we attach to those feelings. The way we interpret our emotions — especially during stressful moments — can either reinforce negative patterns or help us grow with more self-awareness and compassion.

Below is a sample Emotional Thought Tracker tailored for healthcare professionals. It offers examples of how common emotions might show up during our clinical work, the kinds of automatic thoughts that can often accompany them, and gentle reframes that can help shift our internal dialogue toward resilience, clarity, and self-kindness.

As you explore it, I encourage you to reflect on your own experiences and consider building your own Emotional Thought Tracker. Personalising it with situations you encounter regularly can be an incredibly powerful tool — giving you a ready-made guide for navigating tricky moments with more confidence, understanding, and emotional balance and helping you build your self-awareness.

Below is a sample of an Emotional Thought Tracker tailored for healthcare professionals to help you get started.

Emotion	Typical Thought in Healthcare Context	Helpful Reframe for Self-Compassion
Anger (Frustration)	"My patient should just trust me and follow the plan."	"It's normal for patients to have fear and questions. I can guide them with patience."
Anxiety (Worry, Fear)	"If I miss something, I'll fail my patient and my team."	"I care deeply about doing a good job, and I can trust my training and processes."
Guilt	"I'm running late again — I'm letting everyone down."	"I'm doing my best. Sometimes things are outside my control, and I can reset with my next patient."
Sadness (Disappointment)	"I wish I could have done more to help that patient."	"It's okay to feel sad — it means I care. I can learn and keep showing up with compassion."
Shame	"If I make a mistake, I'm a bad clinician."	"Mistakes don't define me — they're opportunities to grow, learn, and improve my practice."
Overwhelm	"There's too much to handle — I can't keep up."	"I'll focus on one task at a time. I don't have to do everything perfectly to make a real difference."

Remember: emotions often overlap. You may experience several of these at once, and that's normal. The goal isn't to "eliminate" emotions, but to understand and manage them with compassion and skill.

3.2 Recognising and Managing Emotional Triggers

"Emotion, which is suffering, ceases to be suffering as soon as we have a clear picture of it."

— Benedict Spinoza

UNDERSTANDING EMOTIONAL TRIGGERS

An emotional trigger is like an iceberg, with only a small portion visible above the surface, while a vast array of memories, experiences, and feelings lie hidden below. In healthcare, where high-stakes decisions are routine, recognising these triggers is a valuable and necessary skill. Building self-awareness means looking beneath the surface to understand the subconscious reactions we experience to certain words, actions, or situations that lead to stress, frustration, or even burnout. Emotional triggers — whether rooted in anxiety, stress, trauma, or anger — often ignite strong responses regardless of a person's current mood. When we understand what sets us off and why, we can learn to pause before reacting, choose our responses with intention, and show up more calmly and compassionately — not just for our patients and team, but for ourselves.

Understanding your emotional triggers isn't just about regulating your own responses though; it's also about influencing the emotional atmosphere around you. When you become aware of how your emotions affect your team or patients, you can choose to respond thoughtfully, which can help foster a more positive environment for everyone involved. This awareness of our emotional landscape is the first step in creating a supportive, healing environment that extends beyond individual reactions.

MAPPING YOUR EMOTIONAL LANDSCAPE

Imagine receiving pointed feedback from a patient's family member that stirs up a strong reaction within you — a flash of frustration or maybe a sting of hurt. That response is a signal, illuminating deeper, often unexamined and subconscious feelings. It may connect to your values, a past experience, or even an underlying fear of not meeting expectations. To manage these moments effectively and appropriately, we need to map out our emotional landscape, identifying the triggers that prompt intense responses. Doing this involves some introspection — taking the time to reflect on our personal values, beliefs, and experiences that shape how we respond to healthcare's unique stresses. Let's uncover how to do this.

<u>A Practical Framework:</u>

When you feel a strong emotional reaction, walk through this process:

1. **Notice the Emotion**
    - What are you feeling? Try naming it (e.g. frustration, guilt, overwhelm). Pay attention to physical cues — tight chest, clenched jaw, shallow breath.

When you have an unexpected or extreme reaction to a situation, take note of the emotions you're experiencing, and any physical sensations present in your body. Recognising a trigger itself is challenging, but paying attention to what you feel in the moment is easier. When a strong emotion arises, consider what you're feeling and label the emotion. Are you frustrated, sad, or anxious? What physical responses accompany it — is your heart racing, are you tense? This awareness can help pinpoint the event that triggered your response.

2. **Identify the Trigger**
    - What event or interaction brought this up? Was it a specific phrase, situation, or person? Was there something familiar about it?

Once you're aware of your emotions, try to walk back through what led to this moment. What were you doing right before feeling this way? Was there a specific moment when the feelings began?

3. **Reflect on the Deeper Story**
    - Ask: "What am I telling myself right now?" You may uncover core beliefs like: "I have to be perfect" or "I'm not good enough."

Triggers often connect to past experiences, so the response may not always "make sense" in the present. For example, a seemingly minor comment might bring up a memory or an association from as far back as your childhood that impacts your reaction.

4. **Pause Before Reacting**
    - Take a breath, step out if needed, or use a grounding technique (such as feeling your feet on the floor). This space creates choice between stimulus and response.

By recognising your emotional responses and taking a brief pause, you create a choice between reacting instinctively and responding thoughtfully. This moment of pause is essential to acknowledging your emotions without judgment. When we give ourselves permission to simply notice our emotions and allow them to be without assigning value or guilt to them, we lay the foundation for healthier emotional regulation.

5. **Debrief with Curiosity**
    - Afterward, reflect on what helped or hindered. Use this insight to update your Emotional Trigger Map (discussed below) with strategies that support you.

Don't feel discouraged if you can't identify a trigger on the first try. Emotions are complex, and it often takes time to untangle them. It's normal to go through this process multiple times before gaining clarity. And if identifying triggers continues to be difficult, professional support from a mental health provider can be valuable.

By recognising your emotions and taking a moment to understand them, you gain the clarity needed to respond with intention, rather than reacting on impulse. This creates the mental space necessary for thoughtful and emotionally intelligent choices in the face of high-stress situations.

STRATEGIES FOR ACKNOWLEDGMENT WITHOUT JUDGMENT

The acknowledgment of emotional triggers must be approached with a spirit of non-judgment. It involves observing reactions as they occur, recognising them for what they are — natural responses to stimuli, rather than indications of professional inadequacy. Mindful acknowledgment means recognising your feelings without labelling them as 'good' or 'bad.' This process allows you to regain control and refocus, ensuring that your responses align with your values rather than an automatic emotional reaction. For example, during a challenging tooth extraction that's taking longer than expected, you might find yourself getting frustrated, being short with or snapping at your dental assistant, or becoming mentally scattered. In this situation, it can help to pause and make an excuse to step out briefly, perhaps to retrieve a particular instrument. This quick break allows a moment to rest your eyes, calm your mind, and reset. Often, I've found that after taking this pause, I return with a clear head, and the procedure that felt impossible only minutes before is completed smoothly and swiftly. Similarly, in a tense situation, simply taking a few deep breaths can defuse the moment, allowing you to choose calmness instead of reacting impulsively. This practice not only prevents the escalation of stress but also models emotional regulation for colleagues and patients alike.

After the fact, it's good practice to reflect on the emotions you experienced — what triggered your reaction, how you responded in the moment, and whether that response helped or hindered the situation. Ask yourself: *What went well? What didn't? What could I do differently next time?* This type of reflection builds emotional awareness over time, helping you not only manage your reactions more effectively but also enhance your emotional intelligence, which is essential for creating stronger relationships and fostering a positive work environment. Like any skill, emotional regulation gets easier the more we practise it — especially when we commit to learning from our missteps with curiosity rather than criticism. When we regulate our emotions with intention, we not only improve our own responses but also create a more supportive and calmer environment for our teams and patients. This positive emotional climate can enhance collaboration and trust, making it easier to navigate even the most challenging situations.

THE RIPPLE EFFECT: EMOTIONAL CONTAGION IN CLINICAL SETTINGS

The concept of emotional contagion, the unconscious mimicry and transmission of emotions between individuals, plays a significant role in healthcare environments. A stressed and anxious healthcare team can inadvertently create a tense atmosphere, influencing patient mood, cooperation, and even their physiological responses. Research suggests that emotions, especially negative ones, are contagious because of nonverbal cues — facial expressions, posture, and tone of voice. For example, when a team member exhibits stress or frustration, it can unconsciously affect others, lowering the overall emotional tone of the room. Conversely, a team that maintains a calm and positive demeanour can foster an environment of trust and support, which is conducive to both patient recovery and team collaboration.

Recognising the power of emotional contagion compels us as healthcare professionals to be mindful of our emotional state and its potential impact on others — whether it's a colleague or a patient. The energy we bring into a room matters. A simple smile, a kind word, or an open posture can transform a tense situation into a positive one.

CREATING A POSITIVE EMOTIONAL ENVIRONMENT

Creating a positive emotional environment begins with small, deliberate actions by each team member and gradually becomes a shared culture that everyone contributes to. A genuinely upbeat tone of voice, a kind word in moments of stress, and sincere expressions of appreciation go a long way in setting the right tone for a healthcare setting. In my practice, I find these seemingly simple interactions essential — they can ease patient anxieties, improve team morale, and, in turn, lead to better overall patient experiences.

The physical environment also has a profound impact on emotional well-being. Bright, welcoming spaces, thoughtfully arranged seating, and artwork or natural elements like plants create a calming ambiance, subtly reinforcing a sense of care and comfort. Whether patients are waiting for appointments or team members are recharging between patients, these small details help foster an atmosphere that feels inviting rather than clinical.

Creating this atmosphere isn't just about managing appearances; it's about cultivating a workplace where positivity naturally thrives. In fact, I consider a positive attitude and an uplifting work environment so vital that I emphasise this point when interviewing potential team members. I look for traits that suggest optimism and a proactive approach to challenges, knowing that a positive mindset not only supports our team but ultimately helps our patients feel at ease.

CREATING YOUR PERSONAL EMOTIONAL TRIGGER MAP

A powerful tool you can use to better understand and regulate your emotional responses is the creation of an Emotional Trigger Map. This simple, practical visual exercise involves:

1. Listing common stressors or scenarios you might encounter in your healthcare setting (or personal life).
2. Identifying the emotional responses they tend to evoke.
3. Brainstorming coping strategies or proactive steps you could take to mitigate their impact.

Your Emotional Trigger Map becomes a personal guide — a living document that evolves with you. By reviewing and updating it regularly, you'll strengthen your self-awareness, build healthier emotional habits, and foster greater resilience even in high-stress environments.

I encourage you to adapt the examples of triggers listed in the table below to suit your own experiences. Add two columns reflecting the emotional responses you notice in yourself to these triggers and potential coping strategies you could use. Over time, you might even create different versions — for work, for home, or for particularly challenging situations you encounter.

Trigger Category	Examples of Common Triggers
Environmental Triggers	• Overcrowded or chaotic clinic atmosphere • Constant background noise or interruptions • Unfamiliar workspaces • Sudden changes to routines or rosters
Workplace or Clinical Triggers	• High-stakes procedures • Time pressures and unrealistic workloads • Receiving unexpected patient complaints • Conflict or miscommunication with colleagues
Personal Life Triggers	• Family stress or caregiving responsibilities • Financial uncertainty • Major life transitions (moving house, becoming a parent, relationship changes
Social and Interpersonal Triggers	• Difficult conversations with patients or team members • Feeling dismissed or undervalued • Fear of judgement during performance reviews or team meetings
Internal Triggers	• Perfectionism or fear of making mistakes • Negative self-talk after a difficult day • Overthinking decisions or outcomes • Fear of disappointing others
Trauma-Related Triggers	• Patient cases that mirror past personal trauma • Anniversaries of stressful events • Exposure to emotionally confronting situations or patient loss
Media and Information Triggers	• Distressing health news • Negative comparisons on professional networking platforms • Information overload from constant alerts, emails, or updates
Health and Wellness Triggers	• Lack of sleep or poor sleep quality • Skipping meals during busy days • Relying on caffeine or sugar for energy • Neglecting exercise or time outdoors • Not drinking enough water

Pro Tip:

Adapting the above table to create your own Emotional Trigger Map can be a powerful way to deepen your self-awareness. This tool helps you pre-emptively plan for moments of emotional strain. As you build your own Emotional Trigger Map, don't just list the triggers — pair each one with a coping strategy you can try when it arises.

Examples could include:

- *Taking three slow, deep breaths before responding*
- *Requesting a 5-minute reset break after a difficult encounter*
- *Journaling a few thoughts at the end of a stressful day*
- *Reaching out to a mentor, friend, or colleague for debriefing*
- *Going for a 10-minute walk outside to clear your head*

These simple strategies can be lifesavers in high-pressure moments. The more prepared you are, the more confident and grounded you'll feel when the inevitable challenges of healthcare, and life in general, arise.

3.3 The Power of Reflection: Learning from Every Interaction

> *"The object of reflection is invariably the discovery of something satisfying to the mind which was not there at the beginning of the search."*
>
> — Ernest Dimnet

THE POWER OF REFLECTIVE PRACTICE

Reflective practice is something I've found to be an incredibly powerful tool for growth — not just professionally, but emotionally as well. It's more than just thinking back on your day or replaying a tricky moment with a patient in your mind. True reflective practice means taking a conscious pause to look at how we responded in certain situations, why we responded that way, and what we might learn from it. Whether it's an interaction with a patient, a team member, or even something we observed in someone else, every moment holds the potential to teach us something — if we're paying attention.

At its core, reflective practice is about being honest with ourselves. True reflective practice means looking at our thoughts, feelings, and actions with curiosity, not judgment. It's not about identifying flaws but recognising opportunities for growth, allowing ourselves the grace to improve with every experience. For those of us working in health-care, our days are full of complex encounters — each layered with emotions, personalities, pressures, and expectations. By taking the time to unpack these experiences, we can start to spot patterns in how we react, where our triggers lie, and how we can strengthen our communication and emotional responses. It helps us better balance empathy with objectivity and ultimately allows us to show up more fully for our patients and teams. It's not about being perfect — it's about getting better, one moment of reflection at a time. Reflection is truly effective when it drives change. It's essential to take the insights gained from reflection and apply them to future interactions. Whether that means adjusting our approach, improving communication, or managing our emotional triggers, reflection should fuel intentional action.

Early in my career, I often found myself getting frustrated when trying to place matrix bands during a filling. The more frustrated I became, the harder it seemed to get the job done. I would go through countless bands, struggling to make it work, only to find myself in a cycle of frustration. After reflecting on these moments, I realised that my emotional state was clouding my ability to think clearly and assess the situation effectively. I learned that I needed to stop, calm down, and give myself a moment to regroup. When I did this, I was able to approach the task with a clearer mindset, and it became much easier to place the matrix band. This experience reinforced for me that reflection isn't just about evaluating the outcome — it's about understanding how my emotions influence my performance and learning to manage them in the moment. Over time, I practiced this approach, and it became second nature, improving both my efficiency and my emotional regulation in clinical settings.

REFLECTION AS A TOOL FOR GROWTH

Integrating reflective practice into our daily routines can be a transformative strategy for enhancing emotional intelligence. One effective approach is to implement a structured reflection at the end of each day or after significant patient interactions. This can take the form of a quiet moment of introspection, a written journal entry, or a discussion with a trusted colleague. In this reflective space, ask yourself these critical questions: "What emotions did I experience during this interaction? How did these emotions influence my behaviour? What can I learn from this experience? What did I do well/what went well? What could I do better or do differently next time?". It can also be helpful to ask for feedback from trusted team members, especially after complex or difficult patient interactions. Sometimes we're either being too hard on ourselves, or we might be missing something that could be improved — an outside perspective can offer valuable clarity that we just can't access when we're too close to the situation. A bit of honest, constructive feedback can shift how we see things, helping us grow and show up better next time. Asking for feedback from colleagues can sometimes feel vulnerable, but it's a powerful tool for growth. When we approach feedback as an opportunity for improvement — rather than criticism — it shifts the focus to collective learning. By welcoming both positive and constructive feedback, we create an environment where everyone can grow and learn from one another. Approach your team with openness and humility, inviting them to share their observations, and be receptive to both the positive and the constructive feedback they offer. By systematically addressing these queries, we can begin to trace the contours of our emotional landscapes, identifying triggers, biases, and areas for growth.

More recently, I had a conversation with one of my associate dentists who had a patient return for the second part of their periodontal treatment. She had decided to check on the work she did during the first appointment by taking an x-ray. Upon reviewing the x-ray, she realised she hadn't removed all the deposits, which meant she needed to redo part of the treatment. When she shared this with me, I reflected on my own approach and told her that, for cases with significant buildup, I always take an x-ray during the same appointment to check for any missed areas while the patient is still numb. This way, I can ensure everything is thoroughly addressed before the patient leaves. She was very receptive to the feedback, and it reinforced the idea that reflection can not only improve our own practice but also help us mentor and support our colleagues, ultimately enhancing patient care.

THE ONGOING JOURNEY OF REFLECTIVE PRACTICE

Reflective practice, therefore, offers a framework for continuous learning and adaptation by prompting us to consider not only what could have been done differently but also what was done well – as touched on earlier. This balanced perspective nurtures a sense of accomplishment and motivates ongoing personal and professional development which is critical in healthcare. Furthermore, by recognising and celebrating moments of successful empathetic engagement or effective communication, we reinforce positive behaviours and strategies, embedding them more deeply into our practice until they become second nature.

The benefits of reflective practice extend beyond personal growth, influencing the very essence of patient care. As we become more attuned to our emotional reactions and more skilled in managing them, we naturally cultivate a more empathetic, relationship-centred approach to the care we provide. This enhanced empathy not only improves patient-provider relationships but also contributes to more accurate diagnoses, tailored treatment plans, and improved patient outcomes. The reflective practitioner, armed with a profound understanding of self and a heightened awareness of others, navigates the complexities of healthcare with grace, compassion, and an unwavering commitment to excellence.

Just as individual emotional regulation can impact patient care, collective reflection within a team can shift the emotional tone of your work environment. Sharing insights with colleagues deepens your collective emotional intelligence, improving the overall emotional climate for both staff and patients. Group reflections, facilitated discussions, and shared learning sessions offer a platform for us to exchange perspectives with others, challenge assumptions, and collaboratively explore solutions to common challenges. This collective inquiry, for example debriefing with the team after particularly complex or difficult patient interactions, not only fosters a culture of openness and support but also amplifies the learning potential of reflective practice, enriching the professional environment with a diversity of insights and experiences.

The journey of reflective practice is ongoing and ever-evolving, requiring sustained effort, a commitment to self-improvement, and a willingness to embrace change. But the rewards are worth it. Reflective practice provides space to process emotional highs and lows, offering clarity in the face of complexity. It helps us stay grounded in our values, even when things get busy or emotionally charged. Over time, consistent self-reflection builds resilience, confidence, and a deeper connection to our purpose — helping us show up as the most grounded, compassionate version of ourselves.

JOURNALING TO ENHANCE SELF-AWARENESS

Journaling, almost like a conversation with oneself, gives us a chance to sort through the emotional and mental chaos that often comes with being a health professional. By putting words to our thoughts and feelings, we can make sense of our internal landscape and gain insights into what drives our reactions and decisions — both at work and personally.

Starting a journaling habit doesn't require long hours of writing, and it may seem simple at first — but its impact can be more profound than we initially realise. In fact, many people dismiss or underestimate the value of journaling, thinking it's too time-consuming or unlikely to bring meaningful results. However, over time, journaling can reveal deeper insights and help us build emotional resilience. This is why it's essential to go in with the right perspective. This isn't intended to be just a log of daily events; it's a reflective exercise aimed at unpacking and understanding the layers of emotional responses we encounter. Even just a few minutes at the end of each day — writing about a challenging moment or a success you had — can help reinforce your self-awareness. Begin by setting aside five minutes, and let your thoughts flow naturally. With time, this habit becomes a powerful emotional release, enhancing both personal well-being and professional growth.

One of the most valuable aspects of journaling is its ability to shine a light on our emotional triggers — especially in a high-pressure environment like healthcare, where those triggers can surface regularly and sometimes unexpectedly in full force. When you journal consistently, patterns start to emerge. You might notice a recurring feeling of frustration in certain patient interactions, or that administrative tasks repeatedly leave you feeling overwhelmed or drained. These insights are gold. They point to the areas where you may need to build resilience or adjust your response in order to protect your emotional well-being. Looking back over past entries deepens this awareness even more.

Often, recurring themes will stand out — sometimes uncomfortably so — but they're important to recognise. For example, if you continually find yourself feeling stressed about paperwork or time constraints, that's a signal it's time to reassess your workflow or seek support in that area. Journaling in this way becomes more than just a venting exercise — it's a roadmap for self-awareness, personal development, and meaningful change in both your well-being and your professional interactions.

Journaling also offers powerful therapeutic benefits. Writing things down allows us to process complex emotions and lighten the mental load we carry day to day. It creates a safe outlet for expressing feelings before they build up and resurface in unhelpful ways. Just like the relief that comes from venting to a friend or family member, journaling provides a similar sense of release — the simple act of putting thoughts to paper can make us feel heard, even if it's just by ourselves. This emotional release helps us stay grounded, making it easier to approach each patient interaction with clarity and composure. For those of us working in healthcare, this practice is more than just a personal ritual — it's a tool that helps us maintain emotional balance, protect our mental wellbeing, and ultimately show up as more present, empathetic clinicians.

It's important to note that studies have shown physically writing things down on paper or in a journal is often more effective than typing into a digital device like a phone or computer. While digital journaling certainly has its advantages — it's convenient, quick, and easily accessible — the act of using pen and paper offers distinct cognitive and emotional benefits that are hard to replicate on a screen. When we write by hand, we slow down, allowing our thoughts to unravel more naturally and intentionally. This slower pace promotes deeper cognitive processing, making it easier to absorb and reflect on what we're experiencing, rather than just transcribing a stream of thoughts. Research also suggests that handwriting activates different parts of the brain linked to memory, emotion, and creativity, enhancing our ability to not just record our thoughts, but to truly understand and learn from them.

There's also something inherently grounding and mindful about the tactile experience of pen on paper. The physical movement, the sound of the pen gliding across the page, even the pause to gather our thoughts before we write them down — all of these sensory elements invite us into a state of presence that typing often bypasses. This ritual of writing becomes a kind of anchor, drawing us back into the moment and deepening the reflective process.

Therefore, journaling is not just a self-reflective exercise but an essential form of self-care. The journey of self-discovery and growth through reflection shapes how we engage with others, deepening our empathy and elevating the care we provide.

REFLECTING ON VALUES, BELIEFS AND BIASES

An important aspect of self-awareness is examining the values, beliefs, and biases that guide us. Our core values — such as compassion, integrity, or teamwork — serve as the internal compass that shapes how we react to challenging situations. Reflecting on these values allows us to align our emotions and actions with our deeper sense of purpose, ensuring consistency between what we believe and how we practice. For example, when we feel frustrated or stressed, pausing to ask ourselves, "Is my response aligned with my values?" helps us gauge whether we are acting in a way that reflects our true beliefs or if adjustments are needed to stay in line with what's most important to us.

Values are more than just abstract concepts — they are deeply held beliefs about what matters most in life. These values influence not only the choices we make but also the way we approach and navigate complex situations. In healthcare, where decisions often have profound consequences, aligning our actions with our values fosters authenticity and integrity. When our decisions are guided by what we truly value, we build trust and create a sense of purpose in our professional lives. For example, if a difficult ethical dilemma arises, reflecting on our core values can provide a framework for making a decision that aligns with both our personal beliefs and professional standards.

Equally important is understanding our beliefs. Beliefs shape how we view the world, how we interpret the actions of others, and how we respond to challenges. These beliefs are not always consciously examined but often form the foundation of our emotional responses. For instance, someone who believes in the inherent goodness of others may approach conflict with the assumption that it can be resolved through understanding and compromise. On the other hand, someone who believes that people are generally self-interested may approach conflict with suspicion, potentially leading to defensiveness or distrust. Becoming aware of these beliefs and how they influence our actions is a critical step in developing emotional intelligence. By understanding our beliefs, we open ourselves to cognitive flexibility — the ability to adjust our thinking in response to new information or changing circumstances, which enhances our emotional intelligence.

Alongside values and beliefs, it is essential to recognise our biases. Biases are the unconscious judgments and assumptions we make based on past experiences, cultural influences, or personal preferences. They can distort our perception, leading to unfair or inaccurate assessments of people and situations. For example, confirmation bias may cause us to focus on information that supports our pre-existing beliefs, while ignoring contradictory evidence. Emotional intelligence helps us manage these biases by fostering emotional self-awareness and self-regulation, allowing us to recognise when our biases may be influencing our reactions and decisions. The more aware we are of our biases, the more equipped we are to challenge them and make more objective, fair decisions.

DISCOVERING YOUR VALUES, BELIEFS, AND BIASES

To truly understand our values, beliefs, and biases, we need to take intentional steps toward self-discovery. Begin by reflecting on your life experiences — consider the moments when you've felt the most fulfilled, proud, or happy. What did those moments have in common? What values were present during those times? Identifying these recurring patterns can provide clarity on what truly matters to you. Similarly, think about the people you admire. What qualities do they possess? What values do they seem to prioritise? This can offer insights into the values you wish to embody in your own life.

Journaling, which we've already discussed in detail, can be an effective tool for uncovering values and beliefs. By writing down your thoughts, especially when faced with challenges or tough decisions, you can start to identify underlying patterns in your thinking. Writing value statements can help clarify and internalise your values, making them more tangible and actionable in your professional practice. Seeking external perspectives — whether through discussions with trusted friends, family, or a mentor — can also provide new insights. These conversations allow you to reflect on your beliefs and gain an outside perspective on how they may be influencing your actions. Additionally, engaging with diverse viewpoints can challenge existing beliefs and help broaden your understanding, encouraging more flexible thinking and empathy.

UNDERSTANDING THE INTERPLAY OF VALUES, BELIEFS, AND BIASES

Understanding the interplay between values, beliefs, and biases provides a powerful lens through which we can enhance our emotional intelligence. By reflecting on our personal values, we can make decisions that are not only ethical but also aligned with our deeper sense of purpose. Understanding our beliefs allows us to approach situations with greater empathy and flexibility, while recognising and managing our biases helps us ensure that we interact with others in an open, fair-minded way.

Ultimately, the process of reflecting on our values, beliefs, and biases is a lifelong journey. It requires consistent self-examination, openness to change, and a willingness to adjust our behaviours in alignment with our evolving understanding of ourselves. By making reflection a regular practice, we not only grow as individuals but also improve the quality of care we provide to our patients, strengthening the connections we have with both those we serve and those we work alongside.

3.4 Mindfulness and Staying Present

> *"Do not dwell in the past, do not dream of the future, concentrate the mind on the present moment."*
>
> — Buddha

In the fast-paced world of healthcare, where the days can feel like a blur and calm moments are few and far between, mindfulness isn't just a nice-to-have — it's one of the most powerful tools we have, and it's available to us anytime, anywhere. What makes mindfulness so effective is its simplicity and accessibility. It doesn't require special equipment or a lot of time — just a conscious moment to pause, breathe, and check in with ourselves. Amid the demands and emotional intensity of clinical work, mindfulness helps us stay grounded, present, and connected — not just to our patients, but to ourselves.

Mindfulness, at its essence, involves a conscious focus on the present moment, an acceptance of our current experience without judgment. For us as healthcare professionals, this practice can become a lifeline, enabling us to navigate the emotional whirlpools encountered daily with a sense of peace and presence. The application of mindfulness techniques, even in the briefest of intervals between patient visits or during short breaks, can significantly amplify our self-awareness. And with that heightened awareness comes greater control over our emotional responses — allowing us to better regulate stress, connect more deeply with our patients, and avoid being swept up in the overwhelm. In professions that so often demand we give to others, mindfulness offers a way to stay centred and refill our own cup, so we can continue to show up with clarity, compassion, and purpose.

Introducing mindfulness into our routine does not need to be a cumbersome addition. Simple exercises, seamlessly integrated into each day, can yield profound benefits. One such technique is the practice of focused breathing, a method that requires nothing more than a moment and the willingness to be still. In the space of a few breaths, we can centre ourselves, drawing our attention away from the chaos of our environment to the rhythm of our own breathing. This act, though brief, acts as a reset button, clearing the mind, calming the heart, and preparing us to face the next challenge with renewed focus and calm.

BREATHING EXERCISES

A common objection to taking a moment to breathe is the perceived lack of time, especially in the middle of a busy day with back-to-back appointments. But I'd argue that we don't have the time *not* to take a minute for a quick breathing exercise. Grounding ourselves in the moment prevents stress from building and allows us to approach each patient with fresh focus. By allowing a moment to reset, we can approach each person and task with fresh attention and calm, keeping our energy — and the environment around us — positive and balanced. These exercises can be done before or after patient interactions, during short breaks, or whenever you feel the need to reset. A few moments of focused breathing can dramatically change the way you approach the next task or patient.

Here are a few simple, effective breathing exercises that can be done quickly and provide a powerful reset:

Box Breathing: This technique is especially helpful for calming the nervous system and reducing stress.

- Inhale for a count of 4.
- Hold your breath for a count of 4.
- Exhale for a count of 4.
- Hold the exhale for a count of 4.
- Repeat for 4–5 cycles. This structured, rhythmic pattern brings a sense of stability and focus, ideal for moments when you feel stressed or overwhelmed.

4-7-8 Breathing: This exercise is great for slowing down your heart rate and can be especially useful at the end of a particularly challenging day.

- Inhale quietly through the nose for a count of 4.
- Hold your breath for a count of 7.
- Exhale completely through the mouth for a count of 8, creating a whooshing sound.
- Repeat the cycle up to 4 times. This slower pattern helps release tension and can also improve sleep quality if practiced before bed.

The Physiologic Sigh: This technique is a simple, science-backed breathing technique that's especially useful when you're feeling overwhelmed or need to combat acute stress and reset quickly.

- Take a deep breath in through your nose, filling your lungs as much as you can. Then, once your lungs feel full, take a second short, sharp inhale to really stretch and expand the air sacs.

- Exhale slowly and fully through the mouth, allowing your body to soften and relax as you release the breath.
- Repeat this pattern 2–3 times. The physiologic sigh rapidly lowers stress by activating the parasympathetic nervous system, helping us calm down almost instantly.

Incorporating these exercises into our day, even if just for a couple of minutes, can help us regain clarity, maintain calm, and ensure we're truly present for each patient or task. These brief pauses are not just for our own well-being — they benefit the entire environment we work in, ultimately contributing to a more positive and focused patient care experience.

MINDFUL OBSERVATION: ANCHORING YOURSELF IN THE PRESENT

While breathing exercises provide a quick reset for the body and mind, mindfulness can also be practiced in a more focused, sensory way through mindful observation. This technique allows us to anchor ourselves in the present moment by observing one simple thing in our environment. What I love about this technique is that you can do it anywhere — no special equipment, no need to sit cross-legged on a cushion with incense burning. You simply pick a single point of focus. That could be the flame of a candle, the feeling of your breath moving in and out of your nose, an object in the room, the hum of a nearby air conditioner, or even the texture of your clothes against your skin. The point is to anchor your attention on one thing and really notice it. Observe every detail you can: the colour, shape, sound, movement, sensation, or rhythm. And as other thoughts or distractions naturally pop into your mind — which they will — don't try to fight them off or judge yourself for losing focus. You just gently bring your attention back to your chosen focal point, over and over.

One helpful way to visualise this practice is to think of your mind like a snow globe that's just been shaken — thoughts swirling everywhere.

Mindful observation is like setting that snow globe down and watching as everything settles. You're not trying to stop the thoughts; you're simply letting them pass by without getting caught up in them. You're observing, not reacting. It's a small practice, but one that can make a real difference in a busy clinical day so you can show up to the next interaction feeling a little more grounded and present.

The benefits of mindfulness extend far beyond the immediate calm it provides. Its consistent practice aids us in staying present, a quality that enhances the delivery of compassionate care. In the midst of back-to-back appointments and the relentless pressure to perform, mindfulness serves as an anchor, ensuring that each patient interaction is approached with a fresh perspective and undivided attention. This presence not only improves the quality of care but also enriches the interaction for both patient and provider, creating a space where genuine connection can flourish and a greater sense of personal fulfilment and professional satisfaction. Although mindfulness exercises only take a few moments, over time, the consistent practice of being present can profoundly alter the way we respond to stress. It strengthens our emotional resilience, making us less reactive to the inevitable challenges of healthcare work, and helps build a long-term sense of inner peace and stability.

MINDFULNESS FOR STRESS MANAGEMENT

Mindfulness encourages a shift in perspective, helping us see stressful situations not as threats but as challenges to be navigated with skill and patience. By activating the parasympathetic nervous system, mindfulness reduces the body's physiological stress response, lowering cortisol levels and creating a sense of calm even in difficult moments. This reframing can dramatically reduce the physiological and psychological impacts of stress, preserving both well-being and the capacity to care deeply for others. Mindfulness practices foster a resilience that buffers against the fluctuations of healthcare work, ensuring that we as professionals remain not just effective but also emotionally and mentally healthy.

Mindfulness doesn't just help in the moment; its consistent practice leads to lasting benefits. Over time, it strengthens our emotional resilience, helping us navigate stressful situations with greater calm and patience. It also helps reduce the long-term impact of chronic stress, preserving our emotional and mental health, and ensuring we continue to provide compassionate care. By integrating mindfulness into our daily routines, we not only enhance our personal well-being but also foster a positive, cohesive work environment. Our calm presence can create a ripple effect, positively influencing our colleagues and patients, leading to better outcomes, stronger team dynamics, and greater professional fulfilment for everyone involved.

3.5 The Role of Feedback in Self-Awareness

"The first step toward change is awareness. The second step is acceptance."

— Nathaniel Branden

Feedback is the mirror through which we can truly see the impact of our emotional responses and interactions. It gives us the chance to refine our approach, elevate patient care, and strengthen the bonds within our teams. At its core, feedback bridges the gap between our perception and reality. It provides a clear view of our professional demeanour as seen by peers and supervisors. This external perspective is invaluable, revealing aspects of our practice that might otherwise go unnoticed. It sheds light on our communication styles, the subtleties of our emotional expressions, and the unintended effects our actions may have on patients and colleagues. The insights we gain from feedback provide a foundation for understanding our emotional landscape and how it shapes the environment we create for those we serve.

CULTIVATING A FEEDBACK-RICH CULTURE

Cultivating a feedback-rich culture within healthcare teams requires a climate of trust, where open dialogue is encouraged. Fear of judgment, reprisal, or inadequacy often stifles honest exchange. Instead, feedback should be seen as a tool for growth rather than a form of criticism. This supportive environment encourages team members to proactively seek feedback and frame requests with specificity, asking for insights into communication, decision-making under stress, or collaboration. Building a feedback-rich culture involves creating safe spaces for feedback exchange. This could include regular check-ins, debriefs after challenging cases, or fostering an open-door policy where team members feel comfortable sharing thoughts and observations without fear of judgment.

When we take the time to build genuine, trusting relationships with our patients, we open up even more opportunities for meaningful feedback. By fostering a sense of openness, we encourage patients to be honest with us — not just about their own experiences with us as individual clinicians, but also about their interactions with the wider team. This feedback provides us with valuable insight into how we're collectively meeting their needs and helps us continuously refine the care we deliver together.

One long-term patient called after her routine check-up to let me know she wasn't happy with how rushed the appointment felt. We booked her in to come back, and when she arrived, she said, "I figured you'd appreciate me being honest with you and letting you know how I felt." And she was absolutely right — I was genuinely grateful. I appreciated her honesty because it gave me the opportunity to make things right and showed that she felt safe enough to speak up. Without that trust, she could have easily gone elsewhere, and we might have never known why.

More recently, another long-time patient came in extremely upset after a miscommunication with our new receptionist. She'd broken a front tooth and wasn't offered an urgent enough appointment, which meant she had to attend a family wedding with her tooth still broken. On top of that, she was supposed to receive a call back to clarify whether the repair would be covered under warranty, and that never happened. She was understandably furious. But because we already had a strong relationship, I was able to listen, apologise sincerely, and make things right. She left feeling heard, supported, and still loyal to our practice. But I know that if that trust hadn't already been there, the situation could have ended very differently — with her walking out for good and likely warning others to steer clear of us.

It's moments like these that remind me just how important it is to invest in building rapport and trust right from the start. Trust isn't built overnight — it takes time, consistency, and care — but it can be broken in an instant. And when it is, emotional intelligence becomes essential. We're all human and mistakes are inevitable, but what really defines us as professionals is how we respond when things go wrong — owning our part, repairing the relationship, and doing better next time. When patients feel genuinely cared for, they're far more likely to give us honest feedback — and with that comes the invaluable chance to learn, grow, and improve the care we provide.

RECEIVING FEEDBACK WITH GRACE

The art of receiving feedback with grace and openness is, in itself, a skill to be honed. Receiving feedback with grace involves more than hearing the words; it requires us to listen carefully, reflect on what's shared, and separate our emotions from the critique, even when it's uncomfortable. When we can view feedback as an opportunity to grow, rather than a personal attack, it becomes a tool for development. For instance, if a colleague provides feedback on your communication style, instead of becoming defensive, you might say, 'Thank you for pointing that out. I hadn't considered that aspect. Can you give me an example of how I can improve?' This approach shows openness and a commitment to improving. A helpful strategy is to take a deep breath before responding, allowing ourselves a brief moment to process the feedback without reacting impulsively. This gives us the space to reflect on the feedback's value and respond with openness, rather than defensiveness.

However, to do this well, we also need to develop a strong sense of self-worth. Without that inner foundation, even the most constructive critique can feel threatening. Building self-worth isn't about ego or perfectionism — it's about acknowledging our strengths, accepting our imperfections, and recognising that we are always a work in progress. With this mindset, feedback becomes less about being "right or wrong" and more about learning and evolving. Receiving feedback is not a passive act; it becomes an active process — asking questions, seeking examples, and engaging in dialogue about how our emotional responses shape our professional behaviour.

Integrating feedback involves more than just acknowledging it; it requires turning insights into action by formulating a plan and setting clear, achievable goals for improvement. You may find it beneficial to delineate specific areas for development, setting realistic, measurable goals that can guide your journey toward enhanced emotional intelligence. For instance, feedback highlighting a tendency to respond sharply under stress might lead to the adoption of stress-reduction techniques we discussed earlier or the implementation of a pause-and-reflect strategy before responding. Taking the time to respond thoughtfully rather than reacting impulsively is a hallmark of emotional maturity. It demonstrates self-control and shows respect for others' perspectives, which helps foster an environment of trust and collaboration. Similarly, insights into the impact of our communication style on team dynamics might prompt the exploration of alternative approaches, the practice of active listening, or the participation in workshops designed to enhance interpersonal skills.

The cyclical nature of feedback ensures a continuous process of growth. Each piece of feedback, whether positive or constructive, builds on the last, creating an evolving path toward self-improvement and greater emotional resilience. This dynamic approach fosters an environment where learning is constant, where each day offers a fresh opportunity to put feedback into action. This iterative process not only drives individual development but also strengthens the collective capability of healthcare teams, ensuring that everyone grows together and builds on shared insights. By continuously integrating feedback, we build resilience. As we refine our skills and grow emotionally, we become better equipped to navigate challenges, bounce back from setbacks, and remain focused on our patients and teams.

A culture that embraces feedback as essential for growth signals a commitment to excellence. It encourages emotional intelligence, self-awareness, and empathy, which ultimately leads to better patient care, stronger teams, and a more fulfilling work environment for everyone.

3.6 Self-Assessment Tools for Personal and Professional Growth

> *"Experiencing one's self in a conscious manner — that is, gaining self-knowledge — is an integral part of learning."*
>
> — Joshua M. Freedman

Self-assessment tools are powerful for growing emotional intelligence — they not only help us evaluate where we're at, but also serve as gateways to deeper self-awareness and professional development. These tools are gaining traction in healthcare because they recognise that managing ourselves and connecting with others is just as crucial as our clinical skills in delivering exceptional care. While these tools provide valuable insights, it's important to remember that no self-assessment tool can capture the full complexity of emotional intelligence. They should be used as one part of an ongoing process of self-awareness and growth.

One widely used tool is the Emotional Competence Inventory (ECI), a 360° feedback assessment developed from the work of Dr. Daniel Goleman and Dr. Richard Boyatzis. What makes it useful is that it doesn't just rely on our own perceptions of how we're doing — it incorporates feedback from others around us, giving a more complete picture of how we show up in the workplace. It focuses on key emotional intelligence competencies like self-awareness, self-regulation, empathy, and relationship management. It's the kind of tool that can reveal blind spots or confirm strengths we didn't fully recognise in ourselves.

Another option is the Mayer-Salovey-Caruso Emotional Intelligence Test (MSCEIT), which works a little differently. Instead of gathering feedback or self-reporting, it presents you with objective tasks designed to assess how well you understand, use, and manage emotions. It's more like a problem-solving exercise rooted in real-life emotional scenarios — which is particularly relevant for those of us in healthcare who regularly deal with high-stakes, emotionally charged interactions.

In addition to these tools, the Emotional Quotient Inventory (EQ-I 2.0) is another popular choice. It provides a comprehensive assessment across a spectrum of emotional skills, offering actionable insights into areas ripe for development. The use of tools like the MSCEIT and EQ-I 2.0, when engaged with regularly, allows for a nuanced understanding of one's strengths and areas for growth, laying the groundwork for targeted developmental strategies.

Many healthcare organisations are also developing their own self-assessment tools tailored to their teams and environments. These can be especially useful because they draw on familiar scenarios — like navigating a difficult conversation with a patient's family, managing a miscommunication with a team member, or addressing ethical dilemmas in treatment planning. By reflecting on how we would respond — or how we actually did respond — in these moments, we begin to recognise patterns in our emotional reactions. That awareness gives us the opportunity to adjust and grow.

What matters most, though, is what we do with this information. Making self-assessment a regular part of our professional development can help us build emotional resilience and strengthen our capacity for compassionate care. It might look like setting aside time to review our results, journaling about insights that came up, or speaking with a mentor to unpack areas we want to work on. A mentor can provide guidance, offer external perspectives, and help keep us accountable in achieving our emotional intelligence goals. Group discussions with colleagues can also be valuable for sharing strategies and fostering accountability. Regardless of the method, the key is to approach this process with curiosity, not criticism.

The process of setting developmental goals, informed by the insights garnered from these assessments, marks a critical step in the journey of emotional intelligence enhancement. This process begins with distilling assessment results into tangible objectives — goals that are specific and achievable, such as enhancing empathy in patient interactions or improving stress management techniques. Articulating these goals and crafting a structured plan for achieving them transforms the abstract concept of emotional growth into a concrete path forward. This path, marked by milestones and checkpoints, helps healthcare professionals navigate their development with clarity and purpose.

These tools are not the end goal — they're just the beginning. Self-assessment tools lay the groundwork for continuous growth. As we revisit them regularly and apply what we've learned, we build a cyclical process of self-awareness that evolves with our professional journey. This iterative process, rooted in the principles of reflective practice, ensures that the development of emotional intelligence is not a finite goal but a lifelong pursuit marked by growth, adaptation, and renewal.

By continuously integrating feedback into our practice, we foster emotional growth and maturity. The more self-aware we become, the better equipped we are to support those we care for. In a profession where human connection is fundamental, self-awareness is not just a personal asset — it enhances our clinical practice by allowing us to respond with greater empathy, make thoughtful decisions, and build trust with our patients.

Chapter 4

Emotional Regulation: Staying Centred in the Chaos

4.1 Cognitive Reappraisal: Changing the Narrative

> *"If a problem can't be solved within the frame it was conceived, the solution lies in reframing the problem."*
>
> — Brian McGreevy

In Chapter 3, we explored the importance of self-awareness in understanding and managing our emotions. As healthcare professionals, we are often confronted with emotionally charged situations that challenge both our technical expertise and our emotional resilience. But self-awareness alone isn't enough. In order to effectively navigate the daily pressures and emotional demands of healthcare, we need the ability to regulate our emotional responses. This is where cognitive reappraisal — one of the most powerful tools in emotional regulation — comes into play.

WHAT IS COGNITIVE REAPPRAISAL?

Cognitive reappraisal is not just about recognising our emotions, but about changing how we interpret and respond to those emotions. It's the process of shifting our perspective to reframe challenging situations, enabling us to respond with greater emotional control and empathy. This skill is essential not only in managing personal stress and emotional reactions but also in maintaining the quality of care we provide to our patients and the collaborative environment we foster within our teams.

At its heart, cognitive reappraisal involves a deliberate change in perspective — a shift in how we interpret an emotionally charged event. This could be something as simple as a challenging patient interaction or as complex as an ethical dilemma. For instance, consider an interaction with a patient who responds to a diagnosis with anger and denial. Initially, such a response might trigger frustration or feelings of inadequacy in you as the healthcare provider. However, when viewed through the lens of cognitive reappraisal, the patient's reaction can be seen as a natural, understandable defence mechanism, a part of their journey toward acceptance. This shift in perspective not only mitigates feelings of personal affront but also cultivates a deeper sense of empathy for the patient's experience, reinforcing your commitment to compassionate care.

REFRAMING CHALLENGES AND STRESSORS

The application of cognitive reappraisal extends beyond individual patient interactions to also encompass the broader challenges we face. The high-pressure environment, characterised by long hours, high-stakes decisions, and the constant demand for precision, can erode our emotional resilience. By using cognitive reappraisal, we can reinterpret occupational stressors as opportunities for growth, framing them as part of a meaningful career dedicated to the betterment of others. This re-evaluation fosters a sense of purpose and fulfilment, providing a buffer against burnout and enhancing overall well-being.

THE PRACTICE OF COGNITIVE REAPPRAISAL

The practice of cognitive reappraisal in real-time is both an art and a science, requiring mindfulness and self-awareness. It begins with recognising our initial emotional response, followed by a conscious pause to reflect on the trigger and automatic interpretation of the event. This pause is crucial, as it creates the space needed to consider alternative narratives that are more aligned with a balanced emotional state and our professional objectives. This shift in thinking empowers us to respond more thoughtfully, rather than impulsively, to the challenges we face.

For example, one time early in my career, I received critical feedback from a colleague regarding my approach to a particular case. My initial reaction was defensive, as if my competence was being questioned — a response that's quite common in the early years after graduation, when many of us are still finding our feet in our new roles. However, I decided to take a moment to breathe and reassess the situation. Instead of viewing the critique as a personal attack, I reinterpreted it as an opportunity to learn and enhance my skills. I considered my colleague's perspective and recognised that their feedback could help me refine my approach for future patients. This reframing not only neutralised my initial defensiveness but also turned a potentially tense interaction into a valuable dialogue about best practices in patient care. By embracing this constructive feedback, I not only grew professionally but also contributed to a culture of learning and collaboration within the group practice I was working in at the time.

BENEFITS OF COGNITIVE REAPPRAISAL

The benefits of cognitive reappraisal go far beyond just keeping ourselves calm in the moment. They ripple outward, influencing the way we show up for our patients, our colleagues, and even ourselves. In patient care, the ability to stay emotionally grounded, especially when things don't go to plan, is crucial. When we can regulate our own emotional responses, we're better equipped to hold space for our patients, even when they're upset, anxious, or fearful. This steadiness fosters trust, creates space for honest communication, and helps patients feel safe and understood — because they can sense we're not reacting to them, but really *hearing* them.

Among healthcare teams, the practice of cognitive reappraisal can help shift the whole culture of a workplace. When individuals learn to pause and reframe setbacks or frustrations, teams are more likely to approach challenges with a problem-solving mindset rather than falling into blame or negativity. It encourages a sense of shared purpose and reduces unnecessary tension. I've seen first-hand how this shift can turn a potentially toxic environment into one where people feel supported, respected, and heard. Over time, these small changes in perspective contribute to stronger relationships, better collaboration, and, ultimately, better outcomes — for both our patients and ourselves.

Moreover, cognitive reappraisal acts as a cornerstone for personal resilience, equipping us with the tools to withstand the emotional ebbs and flows of our chosen path. It provides a framework for processing grief, handling stress, and confronting ethical dilemmas, ensuring that we remain not only functional but also emotionally present and engaged in our work. This resilience has far-reaching implications, contributing to a sustainable career in healthcare and a personal life enriched by a deep sense of purpose and fulfilment. We will delve deeper into building resilience later in this chapter.

4.2 Practical Techniques for Emotional Regulation and Stress Management

---

"Between stimulus and response, there is a space. In that space is our power to choose our response. In our response lies our growth and our freedom."

— Viktor E. Frankl

Being able to find a sense of calm amid the chaos of our world is essential, and simple yet powerful breathing techniques are key to achieving this. These tools serve not just as techniques but as valuable allies that help us reset our internal balance quickly. By using these methods, we ensure that our emotional responses in high-pressure situations are thoughtful actions rather than impulsive reactions. Rooted in ancient practices and supported by modern science, these techniques bridge the body's natural fight-or-flight response with our mind's ability to respond with calmness and clarity.

NAMING AND NOTICING: IN-THE-MOMENT STRATEGIES

Emotional regulation plays a critical role in maintaining the delicate balance between emotional involvement and professional detachment. It's not a passive process — it's an intentional skill that helps us stay grounded in emotionally charged situations. At its core, emotional regulation means learning how to manage our responses so that they align with the needs of the moment, rather than allowing our emotions to hijack our judgement or behaviour. One simple yet powerful technique that supports this is "emotional labelling." This involves identifying and naming the emotions we're experiencing in real time — saying to ourselves, "I'm feeling frustrated" or "I'm feeling anxious." It might sound basic, but it's incredibly effective. By naming what we're feeling, we create just enough space between the emotion and our response to allow for reflection instead of reaction. It breaks the cycle of automatic emotional responses and gives us a chance to choose how we want to move forward.

Another useful strategy is "emotional distancing," which is sometimes misunderstood as emotional detachment. Emotional distancing doesn't mean disconnecting or numbing ourselves — it means creating enough psychological space to see the emotion clearly without being consumed by it. Rather than saying, "I'm angry," we might shift the language slightly to, "I'm noticing that I'm feeling angry" or "I'm noticing feelings of anger." It's a subtle but important distinction. This approach encourages us to adopt the perspective of an observer, which can help us remain calm, collected, and objective — especially in high-stress situations. It gives us a moment to step back and assess: Is this emotion helping or hindering what I'm trying to achieve in this moment?

Practices like emotional labelling and emotional distancing are especially useful in healthcare, where our reactions carry significant weight — not just for our own wellbeing, but for how we communicate, make decisions, and support our patients. They help us approach situations with clarity and compassion, ensuring that our actions are guided by insight and intention, not impulse or overwhelm.

BREATHING TECHNIQUES FOR STRESS MANAGEMENT

The utility of these breathing exercises in healthcare settings cannot be overstated. These techniques are designed to be discreet, requiring no special equipment or environment, making them perfect for the fast-paced and often public arenas where we work. One such technique, the 4-7-8 method, involves inhaling quietly through the nose for 4 seconds, holding the breath for 7 seconds, and exhaling completely through the mouth for 8 seconds. This method, and the others discussed earlier in Section 3.4, can be done during brief lulls between patient consultations or in preparation for a challenging procedure, providing a mental reset that clears the cognitive deck for the tasks at hand.

Another helpful technique is diaphragmatic breathing, also known as "belly breathing." This method engages the diaphragm, encouraging full oxygen exchange, which reduces the heart rate and blood pressure. Diaphragmatic breathing is particularly useful when anxiety or anticipation begins to build, allowing us to return to a state of physiological calmness and mental clarity. The process involves sitting comfortably or lying flat, placing one hand on the belly and the other on the chest, and breathing in deeply through the nose so that the diaphragm expands outward. The exhale, longer than the inhale, is through pursed lips, creating gentle resistance and further promoting relaxation.

The science underpinning these breathing exercises offers a fascinating glimpse into the body's complex response mechanisms to stress. At the heart of this science is the autonomic nervous system, the sympathetic and parasympathetic nervous systems, which regulate unconscious bodily functions. The sympathetic nervous system triggers the body's "fight or flight" response, a necessary survival mechanism but one that can be overstimulated in the high-stress scenarios common in healthcare. Breathing techniques act directly on this system, mitigating its response, and activate the parasympathetic nervous system, often referred to as the "rest and digest" system. This activation initiates a decrease in heart rate and blood pressure, a reduction in stress hormone levels, and a shift toward a calmer, more restored state.

The ability to consciously influence our physiological state through controlled breathing enhances not only stress management but also our ability to engage empathetically and make clear-headed decisions. In emotionally charged situations, this practice allows us to step back, recalibrate, and approach challenges with greater clarity and compassion.

These breathing techniques, when practiced regularly, contribute to a sustained improvement in emotional regulation. Over time, the body begins to associate these breathing patterns with a state of calm, making it increasingly easier to access this state under stress. This conditioning, akin to muscle memory but for the nervous system, enhances our resilience, equipping us with a tool that is both preventative and restorative, ready to be deployed in anticipation of stress or in response to it.

PRACTICING PROGRESSIVE MUSCLE RELAXATION (PMR)

The best techniques for tackling stress blend ancient wisdom with modern science. In addition to breathing techniques, progressive muscle relaxation (PMR) is another effective method for reducing stress. By tensing and then releasing muscle groups, PMR induces a wave of relaxation throughout the body. This practice is a simple yet effective counterbalance to stress, helping to release physical tension and promote overall calm.

To practice PMR, start by finding a comfortable and quiet space, either sitting or lying down. Begin with your feet, curling your toes and tensing the muscles in that area for five seconds while taking a deep breath. Then, slowly release the tension for ten seconds, allowing relaxation to wash over you. Move through the body sequentially, tensing and relaxing other muscle groups like the calves, thighs, hands, arms, back, shoulders, neck, jaw and face. As you practice, pay attention to how the muscles feel when tensed and how your body responds to the release of tension. This method not only alleviates muscle tension caused by stress but also reinforces the connection between mind and body, enhancing overall well-being.

In many ways, PMR shares similarities with Savasana, the final resting pose in yoga, often referred to as "corpse pose." In Savasana, the body remains still while the mind scans and softens each part, bringing awareness to the subtle shifts in sensation, breath, and presence. Just like in PMR, the focus in Savasana is on releasing muscular effort and consciously relaxing the body — bringing stillness and calm to both the body and mind. The difference is that while Savasana is more passive, PMR introduces active tension followed by release, making the contrast more pronounced and, for some, more effective in recognising and letting go of tension. Both practices, however, are incredibly grounding and restorative — especially in the context of busy, high-pressure healthcare environments where stress can so easily take hold.

Creating a relaxing environment with minimal distractions can further enhance the benefits of either practice, helping to anchor you in the present and restore a sense of calm and clarity before stepping back into the demands of the day.

PMR ACTIVITY

Visual Guide: Progressive Muscle Relaxation (PMR)

A simple tool to reset and reconnect — anytime, anywhere.

Step 1: Get Comfortable

- *Sit or lie down in a quiet space.*
- *Close your eyes if you feel comfortable.*
- *Take a deep breath in and slowly exhale.*

Step 2: Focus and Breathe

- *You'll work your way from your toes to your face.*
- *For each muscle group:*
- *Inhale and tense the muscles for 5 seconds.*
- *Exhale slowly and release for 10 seconds, noticing the relaxation.*
- *Pause and feel the difference.*

Step 3: Move Through the Body

- *Feet & Toes – Curl them tightly, then release.*
- *Calves – Flex your feet up, then let go.*
- *Thighs – Squeeze, then relax.*
- *Hands – Make a fist, then open wide.*
- *Arms – Bend your elbows, tense your biceps, then release.*
- *Back – Arch gently, then relax.*
- *Shoulders – Shrug up toward your ears, then let them drop.*
- *Neck & Jaw – Press your tongue to the roof of your mouth, clench your teeth then relax.*
- *Face – Scrunch your face tight, then soften completely.*

Step 4: Finish with Stillness

- *Stay in stillness for a minute or two.*
- *Let your breath return to normal.*
- *Notice how your body feels now compared to when you began.*
- *Gently wiggle your fingers and toes to return to the present.*

Feel the shift? You just gave your nervous system a reset.

VISUALISATION FOR IMPROVED PERFORMANCE

Another powerful tool is visualisation exercises, which involve mentally rehearsing a positive outcome for an upcoming potentially stressful situation. This practice does more than just keep our minds anchored in positivity; it can significantly help us manage stress and enhance performance. By mentally rehearsing challenging scenarios, we can desensitise ourselves to anxiety-provoking situations, allowing us to approach them with greater calm and composure. Visualisation can also boost our confidence. When we mentally practice our responses to high-pressure situations, we reinforce our belief in our abilities and counter negative thoughts (our inner critic) that might otherwise undermine our performance. This increased self-assurance translates to improved performance, as we become better equipped to anticipate challenges and develop effective strategies for overcoming them. Moreover, visualisation helps us set clear goals by solidifying our desired outcomes and making them feel more attainable. As we visualise these goals, our brains activate similar neural pathways as if we were actually performing the tasks at hand. This connection not only enhances our familiarity with the tasks but also builds the neural pathways that facilitate the action we'll be required to take when the time comes.

While these techniques may seem simple to implement, their impact is anything but trivial. They provide a solid defence against the mental and emotional challenges that come with critical decision-making and emergency response, empowering us to navigate these pressures with greater ease and clarity.

PREPARATION AND SCENARIO PLANNING

In the often unpredictable world of healthcare, preparation and scenario planning are two of the most powerful tools we have for staying calm and in control. I like to think of it as rehearsing for a play — you go through the script so many times that, when showtime comes, you don't have to think, you just act. Before any complex or high-stakes procedure, I find it incredibly helpful to run through the entire workflow with the whole team. When everyone understands the sequence, their role, and the plan for managing potential complications, the whole room feels calmer, more focused, and ready to respond if things take a turn.

A great way to reduce stress — and avoid decision fatigue — is by making as many procedures as routine as possible. For example, my workflow for every standard appointment is exactly the same, every single time. Even when I'm doing something as simple as a clean, I use the instruments in the same order and move around the mouth in the same pattern. It might seem small, but this consistency allows my brain to stay one step ahead and helps me reserve mental energy for when I actually need to problem-solve or think quickly on my feet. It also makes things easier for my assistant — when we both know what's coming next, it keeps everything flowing smoothly and efficiently, with less mental strain for everyone involved.

Regular team debriefings after procedures or challenging situations are just as important. They give us space to reflect on what worked, what didn't, and what we can do better next time. When we build in that time for reflection and learning, we strengthen not just our processes, but also our trust and cohesion as a team. So when the unexpected does happen — and it will — we're not scrambling. We're ready, calm, and working together.

BUILDING CONFIDENCE THROUGH COMPETENCE

I've always believed that knowledge equates to power, and skill translates to safety — especially in healthcare. Confidence is built through knowledge and skill. It isn't an innate trait or something that magically appears one day; it's built slowly over time through consistent effort, experience, and a commitment to lifelong learning. Every interaction with a patient, every challenge faced, and every complication encountered offers an opportunity for growth. This ongoing development isn't just about ticking boxes for CPD points — it's about building a solid foundation of competence that allows us to feel calm, capable, and in control under pressure.

Confidence that's grounded in real knowledge and honed skill becomes one of the most powerful antidotes to stress and anxiety. When we feel competent, we're less likely to spiral into self-doubt or panic when something unexpected happens. Instead, we approach challenges with a sense of steadiness and trust in ourselves. That sense of "I've got this" doesn't just benefit us — it directly impacts the way our patients experience care, too. People can feel when they're in capable hands, and that reassurance makes a huge difference to the therapeutic relationship.

Through formal education, clinical experience, hands-on training, and informal exchanges with colleagues, we continue to refine our competence. I can't tell you how many little tips or techniques I've picked up in corridor chats, from posts on online forums or by simply watching a more experienced colleague work. These moments, often small, compound over time to make us more capable and resilient practitioners.

As science and technology continue to evolve, I genuinely believe we have a responsibility to stay up to date. Not just because it makes us better clinicians, but because our patients deserve the best we can offer. Staying current means we're not just reacting to the demands of our work — we're getting ahead of them, equipped with the knowledge, skills, and confidence to make sound decisions, even when the pressure is on. And that's what transforms a potentially stressful situation into a challenge we're ready to meet head-on.

LEVERAGING PEER AND SUPERVISORY SUPPORT

Finally, leaning on peer and supervisory support is one of the most effective ways to protect our emotional well-being. Sharing experiences, venting, or simply debriefing with others can provide the relief and reassurance needed to handle the pressures of healthcare. Whether through informal conversations or structured check-ins, these moments remind us that we are not alone. When we share not just our wins but also the times we felt unsure, overwhelmed, or even defeated, we create a culture where vulnerability is met with empathy rather than judgment. That openness takes courage, but it also strengthens relationships, boosts morale, and encourages others to speak up when they're struggling too.

The most supportive environments I've worked in have always had this undercurrent of "I've got your back." Supportive environments create psychological safety, which encourages openness and fosters growth. When leaders model emotional intelligence by listening openly offering constructive feedback, and checking in with their teams regularly, they create a culture where individuals feel safe to speak up, ask for help and express vulnerability. This open communication strengthens relationships, boosts morale, and combats burnout. We will delve deeply into leadership in the next chapter.

4.3 The True Role of Self-Care in Preventing Burnout

> *"I have come to believe that caring for myself is not self-indulgent. Caring for myself is an act of survival."*
>
> — Audre Lorde

WHY SELF-CARE MATTERS IN HEALTHCARE

In the constant drive to care for others, it's easy to lose sight of our own needs. We walk a fine line between showing up with dedication and slowly edging toward burnout. That's why self-care isn't a luxury — it's a non-negotiable for staying emotionally steady and professionally sustainable. It's a way of saying, "I matter too," and recognising that we can't show up for others if we're running on empty. You really can't pour from an empty cup! I've found this especially true when you're wearing multiple hats — managing a business, running a household, and trying to be everything to everyone. In those moments, the demands on your time and energy multiply and the idea of putting yourself first can feel impossible or even selfish — but it's actually the opposite. Prioritising your well-being isn't just about survival; it's the foundation for doing your best work, being present with your patients, and showing up as your best self in every area of your life.

DESIGNING A SELF-CARE PLAN THAT WORKS FOR YOU

The architecture of a self-care plan should be as personal and intentional as the care we provide our patients. There's no one-size-fits-all — your plan needs to reflect your unique needs, preferences, and lifestyle. At its core, self-care should address the physical, emotional, and social pillars of well-being.

Physical self-care is often the most visible and tangible aspect, but also the one we're most likely to put off when we're tired or busy. The irony is that we don't just wake up full of energy — energy is something we have to create. Movement, even gentle activity, generates energy, boosts mood, and helps us manage stress more effectively. Whether it's a brisk walk, a yoga session, or something more structured, regular exercise — alongside a balanced diet, good sleep hygiene, and proper rest — forms the foundation of physical resilience. These practices don't just support our health — they keep us mentally sharper, more emotionally balanced, and better equipped to handle the daily demands of our work.

Yet, the essence of self-care extends beyond the physical, delving into the realms of emotional and social well-being. Emotional self-care is about intentionally doing things that refill our emotional cup — it's not just about stopping, but about choosing the *right* kind of pause. That's where understanding the difference between rest, relaxation, and recharging really matters.

- Rest is what we need when we're physically, mentally, or emotionally depleted. It's about pausing and allowing ourselves to recover. That could mean taking a proper day off (and truly unplugging), prioritising sleep, or simply listening to your body when it says "enough."
- Relaxation is more active. It helps ease tension in the body or mind — whether that's through a walk in nature, a warm bath, reading a good book, or watching something that makes you laugh. It's about letting go and being present.

- Recharging is the most energising of the three. It's not just about recovery — it's about restoration. This could mean learning something new, doing something creative, connecting with a friend who lifts you up, or helping someone in a way that reaffirms your sense of purpose.

We need all three. Rest helps us recover what's been drained. Relaxation helps us release what we've been holding. And recharging builds us back up so we can return with more to give.

Meditation, mindfulness, or immersing yourself in hobbies that spark joy can offer all three benefits depending on how and when they're used. Emotional self-care isn't a luxury — it's a form of maintenance. Without it, we don't just burn out — we lose our ability to show up as the compassionate, centred professionals our patients need.

Social self-care is equally vital. The cultivation of meaningful relationships acts as a buffer against the isolation that can creep into our work. Whether it's connecting with family, friends, or colleagues in a way that has nothing to do with work, these moments help us recalibrate, feel seen, and return to our roles with renewed energy and perspective

SELF-CARE BUILDS RESILIENCE AND EMOTIONAL INTELLIGENCE

The symbiosis between self-care and emotional resilience cannot be overstated. Engaging in deliberate self-care routines enhances your capacity to manage stress and navigate the emotional complexities inherent in healthcare. This bolstered resilience equips us with the fortitude to face challenging patient interactions, ethical dilemmas, and the fluctuations of our work with a steady heart and mind. It fosters a robustness that allows us to encounter stress, not as an overwhelming force, but as a manageable aspect of our professional landscape, one that can be navigated with wisdom and patience.

The consistent practice of self-care rituals cultivates a heightened level of emotional intelligence, crucial for patient care. A healthcare professional who attends to their well-being is better positioned to approach patient interactions with empathy, patience, and clarity. They possess the emotional bandwidth to truly listen, to empathise deeply with patient concerns, and to communicate with compassion and understanding. This enhanced emotional intelligence not only improves patient outcomes but also contributes to a more rewarding and fulfilling professional experience, where connections with patients and colleagues are marked by authenticity and warmth.

MAKING TIME VS. MAKING EXCUSES

The journey of integrating self-care into our daily routines is not without its challenges. Time constraints, workload pressures, and the unpredictable nature of healthcare work can all serve as formidable barriers. But let's be honest — people often say they don't have time as a way of excusing themselves from doing the things they know they need to do. The truth is, when something really matters to us, we make time for it. So when we say we don't have time for self-care, what we're really saying is that it's not a priority. And that's where the shift needs to happen. The commitment to self-care is a commitment to sustainability in the healthcare profession. It's not a luxury or a treat — it's a non-negotiable. It requires a re-evaluation of priorities and an honest acknowledgment that caring for ourselves is not selfish; it's necessary. It takes discipline, yes, but also self-respect — the willingness to carve out time, even in the chaos, for the activities that nourish our body, calm our mind, and restore our spirit.

CREATING A CULTURE OF WELLBEING IN HEALTHCARE

While self-care is ultimately a personal responsibility, it becomes far more sustainable when supported by the environments we work in. Healthcare institutions have a huge role to play in creating a culture that genuinely values and prioritises staff well-being — not just in theory, but in practice. That might look like policies that support work-life balance, access to mental health resources, or even simply ensuring there's a quiet space to take a proper break during the day. When the workplace encourages and normalises self-care, it sends a clear message: your wellbeing matters. And ultimately, that benefits everyone. Because when we feel supported, cared for, and balanced, we're in the best position to show up fully for our patients and provide the kind of care that really makes a difference. It's that simple.

Reflection: Recharging with Intention

Take a few quiet minutes to reflect on the following questions. You can jot your answers down in a journal, on your phone, or just think them through — whatever feels right for you.

- *What are three activities that genuinely recharge you — not just help you rest, but actually leave you feeling energised or restored?*
- *(e.g., walking outdoors, listening to music, painting, catching up with a friend)*
- *When was the last time you did one of these activities? What got in the way, if anything?*
- *What's one small thing you can prioritise this week to support your physical, emotional, or social wellbeing?*
- *(Try to make it specific and realistic — something you could do even on a busy day.)*
- *Finish this sentence:*
- *"I feel most balanced and capable when I..."*

Tip: Revisit your responses each month. They can serve as a gentle checkpoint to make sure you're staying connected to what fills your cup.

REFILL YOUR CUP: A GO-TO LIST FOR LOW ENERGY DAYS

When we're depleted, our thinking narrows, and it becomes harder to make decisions — even about what might help. That's why having a list like this ready to go is so powerful. It removes the guesswork and helps you reconnect with yourself, one small action at a time. As writer Anne Lamott wisely put it, *"Almost everything will work again if you unplug it for a few minutes, including you."* These small resets are not just indulgent — they're essential. For the moments when you're running on empty and can't think straight, pick one of the small things from the list below — no overthinking required.

To Calm Your Nervous System

- Take 10 slow deep belly breaths.
- Do a short guided meditation (try Headspace, Insight Timer, Aura or YouTube).
- Sit outside and feel the sun or breeze on your skin.
- Place your hand on your heart and take 3 slow breaths.
- Do a 2-minute body scan similar to what we discussed earlier (start at your toes, move upward).

To Shift Your Energy

- Step outside and walk around the block.
- Stretch your arms up and roll your shoulders back.
- Put on music and dance it out — just one song.
- Do a 30-second cold water splash on your face or wrists.
- Change your environment (move to a different room or go outside).

To Nourish Emotionally

- Call or message someone who gets you.
- Re-read a favourite book passage or quote.
- Watch a short video that always makes you laugh.
- Write down three things you're grateful for today.
- Hug your pet, your partner, your pillow — anything warm and soft.

To Reconnect with Joy

- Do something with your hands (paint, bake, garden, doodle).
- Make a cup of tea or coffee and drink it slowly, no distractions.
- Play a song that lifts your mood. Sing your heart out!
- Watch or listen to something that feels uplifting or comforting.
- Spend 5 minutes on a hobby you love (even if it's just for fun or you're still learning).

Save this list somewhere easy to find — bookmark it, take a photo of it, or pin it up near your workspace.

4.4 Balancing Empathy and Professional Detachment

> *"Do not confuse healthy detachment with avoidance. In my opinion, the difference between the two are acceptance and acknowledgment."*
>
> — Robin S. Baker

OVERCOMING EMPATHY BLOCKS

While empathy is often seen as an innate trait, the reality is that it can be disrupted — sometimes subtly, other times dramatically — by a range of internal and external factors. These empathy blocks are common in healthcare, and acknowledging them is the first step toward addressing them with intention.

On a personal level, empathy can be blocked by unconscious biases and assumptions. Whether related to a patient's appearance, cultural background, age, or even perceived compliance, these preconceptions can quietly influence how we engage with and respond to our patients. It might show up as less eye contact, a shift in tone, or even a subtle lack of warmth — all of which a patient will notice, even if we're unaware we're doing it. For example, a clinician may feel less empathetic toward a patient they perceive as non-compliant or difficult, without taking the time to explore the barriers that may be influencing the patient's behaviour. Recognising that we all carry unconscious bias is not about blame — it's about developing the self-awareness to catch ourselves before those biases translate into behaviour that compromises care.

Emotional fatigue is another major empathy blocker, particularly in high-pressure environments where clinicians are expected to deliver high-quality care under immense stress. When you're running behind, overwhelmed, or feeling emotionally spent, it can be difficult to connect with patients on a deeper level. Instead of engaging compassionately, the focus shifts to "getting through the list," and patient interactions can become transactional. This is where burnout and compassion fatigue start to erode not just our own wellbeing, but the quality of care we provide.

BUILDING EMPATHY THROUGH REFLECTION AND TRAINING

One way to address these blocks is through reflective practice. Taking the time — whether formally during supervision or informally during a walk or journaling — to reflect on your interactions and emotional responses can bring valuable insights to the surface. You might ask yourself: "Why did I find that patient frustrating today?" or "What was I feeling when I walked into that consultation?" This kind of reflection helps us make sense of our emotional reactions and realign with our core values as healthcare providers. It's not about being perfect — it's about staying connected to our purpose and recalibrating when we drift.

Empathy can also be enhanced through specific training in perspective-taking and emotional awareness. Role-playing exercises, simulated patient scenarios, and case-based discussions can help clinicians practice seeing the world through someone else's eyes. Even simple practices like journaling from the perspective of a challenging patient can shift how we engage with them in future encounters.

At an organisational level, workplaces need to create psychologically safe environments that support empathy, not just demand it. When clinicians are unsupported, overworked, and undervalued, empathy becomes just another item on the to-do list. Providing spaces for staff to decompress — quiet rooms, debriefing sessions after difficult cases, or even structured peer support — can make a significant difference. Equally important is ensuring team members feel seen and heard, not just patients. Empathy is contagious; when we feel valued and supported by our teams and leaders, we're much more likely to extend that same care to our patients.

FINDING THE MIDDLE GROUND

We often walk a tightrope between feeling deeply for our patients and maintaining the necessary distance to make clear-headed decisions. Finding this balance is no easy task. It involves a lot of self-reflection and awareness of our own emotional reserves, as well as putting strategies in place to protect both our well-being and the quality of care we provide. Engaging with our patients' stories while also keeping our professional mindset intact is essential for delivering the best outcomes.

The quest for equilibrium begins with the understanding that emotional involvement and professional detachment aren't opposing ends of a spectrum — they're two sides of the same coin in healthcare. We need both. Emotional involvement is what allows us to be empathetic, to form meaningful connections with our patients, and to truly understand what they're going through. It's what humanises the care we give and helps patients feel safe, seen, and supported. But at the same time, a degree of professional detachment is absolutely essential — without it, we risk losing perspective, making clouded decisions, or burning ourselves out entirely.

For those of us who are naturally high in emotional intelligence, this balance can actually be harder to strike. Our ability to sense and respond to the emotions of others is a strength — but it can also become a burden. When we're not careful, we start to absorb the emotional states of the people around us, often without even realising it. This emotional mirroring — where we unintentionally take on a patient's anxiety, grief, or frustration — can leave us feeling emotionally drained or overwhelmed, especially when we're surrounded by distress or high-stakes decisions all day. If left unchecked, this constant internalising of others' emotions can quietly accumulate, eventually leading to stress, fatigue, or even burnout.

That's why it's so important to recognise when we're taking on too much emotionally, and to consciously set boundaries — not to push people away, but to protect our own ability to show up with compassion and clarity. Striking the right balance between emotional attunement and emotional protection allows us to maintain empathy without becoming emotionally saturated. It's about staying connected, without losing ourselves in the process.

SETTING HEALTHY BOUNDARIES

Setting clear boundaries — both emotional and professional — is absolutely essential to finding and maintaining that middle ground. These boundaries are like protective guardrails; they help define how much of ourselves we can give without compromising our wellbeing or professional integrity. But learning where those lines are often takes time and self-awareness. In the early stages of our careers, it's especially common to push past our own limits — whether it's performing a procedure we're not fully confident in because we don't want to appear inexperienced, or giving in to a patient's request for a treatment we know isn't the best option, just to avoid confrontation. We do it with good intentions, trying to prove ourselves or keep patients happy, but over time, that constant override of our internal cues chips away at our confidence and emotional resilience.

Understanding and communicating our boundaries begins with recognising our own triggers, limitations, and values. Once we're clear on those internally, we can start expressing them externally — whether it's calmly explaining why a certain treatment isn't in the patient's best interest, or setting expectations around what we can and can't offer. Importantly, this isn't about distancing ourselves from patients; it's about engaging with empathy while staying anchored in what's clinically appropriate and emotionally sustainable. Boundaries don't diminish our care — they make it more consistent, ethical, and ultimately, more effective. They allow us to show up with compassion and clarity, without burning ourselves out in the process. Boundaries are so important that we will discuss them in more detail in Section 4.6, where we explore how to effectively implement and maintain them in our practice.

4.5 Bending Without Breaking: How We Build Real Resilience

"Life doesn't get easier or more forgiving, we get stronger and more resilient."

— Steve Maraboli

Resilience is like a protective shield, helping us tackle the emotional ups and downs we face every day. It's a quality that's powerful but can always be strengthened. Building resilience means we not only learn to weather the storms of patient care and workplace challenges, but we also find ways to rise above them. Making resilience a priority is key, and it involves putting intentional effort into strategies and practices that boost our ability to adapt and thrive under the pressures of our careers.

CREATING A SUPPORTIVE WORK CULTURE

One of the most powerful ways to build resilience is by creating a positive work environment — somewhere that feels safe, encouraging, and grounded in mutual support. When people feel valued and part of a team that genuinely cares, they're far more likely to bounce back from stress and stay engaged. This doesn't have to mean flashy wellness programs or expensive initiatives. In smaller practices like ours, it can be as simple as acknowledging a job well done, celebrating small wins, or making space for a team coffee break where people can laugh and decompress. Having a culture where people feel comfortable sharing challenges and coping strategies — whether it's through regular catch-ups, debriefs after tough days, or just checking in with one another — can make all the difference. These seemingly small acts build connection, boost morale, and create a sense of shared purpose that helps us weather the tougher days together.

PERSONAL PRACTICES TO STRENGTHEN RESILIENCE

Another powerful way we can build resilience is through simple, consistent practices that strengthen our ability to stay grounded in the face of stress. One of the most effective tools in this space is mindfulness meditation. As we explored earlier in Chapter 2, mindfulness isn't just a trendy wellness buzzword. Mindfulness is really about training ourselves to be present — to bring our awareness to the here and now without judgment. In the whirlwind of healthcare, where we're constantly pulled in multiple directions and emotionally stretched, mindfulness helps us pause, breathe, and anchor ourselves. Over time, this kind of present-moment awareness improves our ability to respond thoughtfully rather than react emotionally, which is crucial when we're navigating high-pressure situations.

One small but powerful habit is using positive affirmations between patient visits. These quiet mental resets — simple phrases like "I am calm and capable" or "I bring care and presence to each interaction" — can shift your mindset in just a few seconds. It's like planting a tiny seed of reassurance that helps anchor you amid the noise. Over time, affirmations like these help create a mental environment where self-belief, steadiness, and purpose can take root and grow.

Resilience workshops are another valuable resource. These are often interactive and practical, offering training in core areas like stress management, emotional regulation, and communication. One of the most beneficial aspects of these workshops is the use of scenario-based or role-play learning. By stepping into simulated versions of difficult conversations or high-stakes moments, we get to practice how we might respond in real life — but in a supportive, low-risk environment. I've found that this hands-on approach not only improves our skills but also boosts confidence, making us feel more capable when faced with similar situations in the real world.

While resilience is often built in the clinical environment, it's also nurtured outside of it. Making time for activities that have nothing to do with work — painting, playing music, hiking, reading, even learning something new — helps reconnect us with who we are beyond our professional roles. These hobbies aren't distractions; they're vital reminders that we are full, multi-dimensional people with interests, creativity, and lives outside of our work. That balance helps keep us grounded, adds joy to our days, and offers perspective when healthcare feels all-consuming.

PURPOSE-DRIVEN GOALS

Another often-overlooked part of building resilience is setting realistic personal and professional goals. In busy clinical environments, it's easy to get caught up in the daily grind and lose sight of the bigger picture. When we take the time to define goals that truly reflect our values and aspirations, it gives our work more meaning. These don't have to be grand, life-altering goals — sometimes, it's about improving how we manage difficult conversations, mentoring a colleague, or protecting time for self-care. The act of striving toward something, even in small increments, helps create momentum and purpose. And when we hit roadblocks — and we will — it's that sense of purpose that keeps us going. The growth we experience as we work through setbacks not only makes us more resilient but also reinforces our belief in our ability to navigate challenges and come out stronger.

TURNING SETBACKS INTO STRENGTH

Resilience isn't about avoiding hardship or pretending everything is fine. It's about acknowledging when things are tough and having the inner strength to move through it without falling apart. In the aftermath of a difficult clinical case, an angry patient interaction, or even a personal setback, resilience gives us the ability to reflect, recalibrate, and return — wiser and more grounded than before. It helps us turn moments of challenge into lessons that fuel our growth. And when we start to see those hard moments not as failures but as part of the journey, that's when we really begin to thrive — not just as professionals, but as people.

Sometimes though, even with the best intentions and strategies, our internal resources aren't enough. That's when turning to professional support — like a psychologist or therapist — can make all the difference. Seeking help is not a sign of weakness; it's a courageous act of self-respect and commitment to our wellbeing. In fact, some of the most emotionally intelligent clinicians I know are the ones who are willing to say, "I need support right now." Because being strong doesn't mean going it alone — it means knowing when to reach out.

And yet, in healthcare — particularly among doctors — there's still a deep stigma attached to seeking mental health support. Many fear that reaching out will jeopardise their careers, compromise confidentiality, or be seen as a weakness in a profession that historically valorises self-sacrifice. As psychiatrist Elissa Ely describes from her work on a physician crisis helpline, doctors in deep distress — those experiencing panic attacks, substance use, depression, or even suicidality — often hesitate to seek formal help. Their most pressing question is not about what treatment might help, but whether the call is truly anonymous. That fear is not unfounded: for years, licensing boards and healthcare institutions have asked intrusive questions about prior mental health care, reinforcing the message that vulnerability could cost a doctor their livelihood.

These structural barriers, combined with the personal and cultural pressures of the profession, contribute to devastating outcomes. Rates of burnout and psychological distress have risen sharply since the COVID-19 pandemic, and the suicide rate among doctors remains alarmingly high. This crisis is not just a personal one — it's systemic, and it impacts the entire healthcare workforce. If we want to create truly sustainable, compassionate systems of care, we must start by dismantling the stigma that prevents clinicians from caring for themselves. Mental health support must become not only accessible, but expected — an integral part of how we train, support, and retain those who care for others. Because healing the healers isn't a luxury — it's a necessity.

F.A.I.L. - FIRST ATTEMPT IN LEARNING

A key component of resilience is how we interpret and respond to setbacks. Our mindset — the lens through which we view challenges — can either erode our confidence or help us grow stronger. That's where reframing comes in. When we shift our perspective on failure, we create space for learning, compassion, and growth. One helpful example is the acronym "FAIL," reimagined as First Attempt In Learning — a powerful reframe popularised by Dr A.P.J. Abdul Kalam, the 11th President of India, who also famously reminded us that "END" stands for Effort Never Dies. When we adopt this mindset, failure becomes feedback, not a final verdict. This is where reframing becomes a superpower.

As Nelson Mandela put it, *"Do not judge me by my success, judge me by how many times I fell down and got back up again."* That mindset — of rising again and again — is what "failing forward" is all about. When we learn to view setbacks as stepping stones, not stumbling blocks, we not only grow individually — we help cultivate a culture where learning, support, and resilience go hand in hand. One where mistakes are embraced as part of the learning curve, not something to be ashamed of.

This simple acronym can be used to help reframe failure with emotional intelligence and self-compassion:

F – Face Your Feelings

Acknowledge any emotions that arise — frustration, disappointment, shame. Consider how the experience may have impacted your sense of self and whether it's reinforcing any negative beliefs you hold about yourself. Don't bury these feelings, and don't let them paralyse you. Processing your emotional response is the first step toward healing and growth. If you feel comfortable, discuss your feelings with someone you trust to help you process the experience, ease the emotional burden and potentially gain a different perspective.

A – Analyse What Happened

Step back and look at the situation objectively. What contributed to the outcome? Were there internal factors, external pressures, or gaps in planning or communication? Try to separate the result from your sense of identity. This isn't about who you are as a person — it's about what happened and what you can learn from it.

I – Identify the Lesson

There's almost always a lesson hidden in failure — if we're willing to look for it. It's also important to recognise failure as a natural part of the journey toward success. What insights can you take away from the experience? What would you do differently next time? When we reframe failure as feedback, it becomes a catalyst for clarity and growth. This mindset not only builds resilience but also transforms setbacks into springboards for deeper learning and personal and professional evolution.

L – Let Go and Move Forward

Mistakes are part of the process. Let go of shame, forgive yourself, and shift your focus forward. See the experience as an opportunity to refine your approach, not as a reason to hold back. Self-kindness here is key — because learning isn't linear, and neither is growth.

THE RESILIENT CLINICIAN

Resilience isn't built in a day — it's cultivated moment by moment, through the choices we make, the way we treat ourselves, and the environments we help create. Whether it's taking a mindful breath between patients, reaching out for support, or reframing a setback with compassion, every small step adds up. The more we practise these skills, the more naturally they become part of who we are. And with that inner strength, we're better able to show up — not just as capable clinicians, but as whole, grounded human beings.

4.6 Boundaries and Avoiding Compassion Fatigue

"When we fail to set boundaries and hold people accountable, we feel used and mistreated."

— Brené Brown

UNDERSTANDING BURNOUT VS COMPASSION FATIGUE

Burnout and compassion fatigue are two of the biggest emotional challenges we face — and while they're often spoken about interchangeably, they're not quite the same thing. Burnout is generally the result of chronic workplace stress — long hours, administrative overload, feeling undervalued or ineffective — which slowly chips away at your motivation, energy, and sense of purpose. Compassion fatigue, on the other hand, is more specific to the emotional toll of caring deeply for others. It often stems from prolonged exposure to patients' pain, trauma, or suffering, and can leave you feeling emotionally drained, numb, or disconnected.

RECOGNISING THE WARNING SIGNS

Both conditions can threaten to erode not only our professional effectiveness but also our personal wellbeing. That's why recognising the early warning signs — like persistent exhaustion, irritability, emotional detachment, physical symptoms such as headaches or muscle tension, or even a growing cynicism towards patients or the job — is so crucial. If you find yourself emotionally drained at the start of each day and dreading heading into work, snapping at colleagues or loved ones, or simply feeling like you have nothing left to give, these are signals from your body and mind that something needs to shift. And the earlier we catch those signals, the easier it is to course correct. Acknowledging the signs without judgement and seeking support — whether through small daily changes or more structured help — is key to regaining balance and protecting both our emotional health and the quality of care we provide.

I know this all too well from personal experience — burnout has been a recurring challenge throughout my career, particularly as a small business owner. The financial pressure and constant responsibility that comes with running a practice, on top of working chairside and delivering patient care, often made it hard to justify taking any time off. For years, I was working six or seven days a week, and even when I did take a day off, the guilt I felt was so overwhelming that it was anything but restorative. It wasn't until I was forced to take a proper break — when I went on maternity leave with my first daughter — that I finally realised how unsustainable my schedule had become. Returning to clinical work just 3.5 days a week, I quickly noticed that I had more energy and enthusiasm, which helped me engage more meaningfully with patients and deliver better care. And interestingly, our revenue even went up. Even after learning that lesson, I still sometimes struggle with the idea of taking time off — and I know I'm not alone. Many of us in healthcare are so driven to help others that we forget to help ourselves. But as we touched on earlier when discussing self-care, you really do need to put on your own oxygen mask first. If we don't look after ourselves, we simply can't give our patients the level of care they deserve.

SETTING BOUNDARIES THAT PROTECT YOU

Finding a sustainable balance between work and life is one of the most important ways we can protect ourselves from burnout — and also one of the trickiest to maintain. The demands of healthcare can blur those boundaries so easily, especially when we care deeply about the people we're helping. But I've learned that setting clear limits around our time and energy isn't just helpful — it's necessary. Prioritising what's truly urgent and important, sticking to realistic work hours, and making time to properly switch off and recharge can make all the difference.

For me personally, having a consistent morning routine sets the tone for my day and helps me feel grounded. Being a morning person, I enjoy getting up early while my family is still asleep. I start by drinking a big glass of water, doing a guided meditation, and reading my gratitude statement. Then, I take my dog for a peaceful walk before returning home to exercise and get everyone else up to start the day. This quiet time in the morning is sacred — it allows me to centre myself and face the day's demands with a calm, refreshed mindset. I'll often repeat affirmations out loud on the drive to work, things like: "Today is going to be a great day. Everything is going to run smoothly. Everyone is going to be happy. The team will not feel stressed. The patients will feel cared for." It might sound simple, but setting that positive intention has a powerful effect on how I show up for the day.

Mindfulness practices like progressive muscle relaxation (PMR) or visualisation exercises, which we discussed earlier, are also incredibly effective tools for preventing burnout and compassion fatigue. I find PMR is best used at the end of the day to help decompress and let go of any tension that's built up. Visualisation, on the other hand, can be really helpful either the night before or the morning of a busy day — mentally rehearsing how I want the day to unfold helps me feel prepared, grounded, and in control.

On the days where I skip my routine — whether I've hit snooze too many times or jumped straight into work mode — I really notice the difference. I feel more reactive, less centred, and my threshold for stress is much lower. It's a reminder of just how important it is to carve out that intentional time for yourself before the day takes over. These small habits are what help me stay present, reduce stress, and show up as my best self for my patients, my team, and my family.

PROTECTING YOUR ENERGY WITHOUT LOSING EMPATHY

It's important to remember that setting emotional boundaries doesn't mean we care any less. In fact, it's quite the opposite. Boundaries are what allow us to keep showing up with empathy day after day, without losing ourselves in the process. They act like a buffer — creating enough space between us and the emotional intensity of the work so we can stay present without becoming overwhelmed.

This doesn't mean becoming cold or detached. It means knowing when to pause and return to our own emotional space, especially after particularly tough cases or conversations. I've spoken to nurses who work in palliative care who've mastered this balance beautifully — they listen with compassion, offer their full presence, and then consciously step back so they can continue supporting the next patient without becoming depleted.

The first step in setting boundaries like this is self-awareness. Noticing when we're feeling more irritable, emotionally numb, or physically tense can help us catch early signs that our reserves are running low. Grounding practices like mindfulness, journaling, or even taking a short walk between patients can help us reset. And sometimes, even light-hearted humour — used gently and thoughtfully — can release tension and protect our emotional reserves without minimising the importance of the moment.

We can't absorb everyone's pain and expect to remain whole. Boundaries are not barriers — they're the scaffolding that allow us to keep doing this work with heart, clarity, and care. Earlier in my career, I found myself crossing my own boundaries more than I'd like to admit — especially in paediatric cases. I remember several situations where I knew a child would be better off receiving treatment under general anaesthetic with a paediatric specialist, but the parents were desperate for me to try treating them in the chair. I could see how hard it was for the family, and I wanted to help — so I said yes, even when I felt in my gut that it wasn't the right call. And every single time, I regretted it. It was traumatic for the child, stressful for everyone involved, and left me emotionally drained. In trying to ease someone else's discomfort, I ended up betraying my own professional judgment and emotional limits. That was a huge lesson for me: boundaries aren't about being inflexible — they're about protecting the wellbeing of everyone involved, including yourself.

BUILDING EVERYDAY TEAM SUPPORT

Support doesn't have to come from a big hospital system or a formal wellness program — it can be built right into the everyday culture of a smaller practice too. In fact, in small teams, it's often even more important. Creating a workplace where well-being is genuinely valued starts with open communication and a willingness to check in on each other — not just about the schedule or the to-do list, but about how people are *actually* doing. It could be something as simple as taking five minutes at the start of the day to check in as a team, or encouraging each other to speak up when things feel overwhelming.

Making mental health resources accessible — whether that's a list of trusted counsellors or creating time for someone to step away for a walk if they need it — sends a strong message that emotional health is just as important as performance. And while we might not have formal peer support groups, we can still create that same kind of space through regular team catch-ups or informal debriefs after challenging days. These little touchpoints go a long way in helping everyone feel seen, supported, and less alone in the tough moments. When people feel safe to be honest about what they're going through, we're much more likely to catch signs of burnout early — and take action *before* someone reaches their breaking point.

SEEKING HELP IS STRENGTH, NOT WEAKNESS

For those already navigating burnout or compassion fatigue, healing takes time — and often, support. Practising self-compassion and gradually re-engaging with work in a supportive, manageable way can be key to progress. Simple actions like taking breaks, setting boundaries, and talking to a therapist or trusted peer can make a meaningful difference. But as we touched on earlier, the hardest step is often admitting we need help in the first place.

In medicine, there's long been a culture of silent endurance. We're trained to push through fatigue, suppress our emotions, and keep going no matter what. It's no wonder that doctors, in particular, are at a significantly higher risk of suicide compared to the general population. Studies have shown that the suicide rate among physicians is more than double that of the general public, with female physicians especially at risk. And yet, many suffer in silence because the stigma of seeking mental health support remains deeply embedded in our profession. We're expected to be superhuman — to juggle unreasonable schedules, emotionally draining cases, administrative pressures, and personal responsibilities, all while presenting a calm and competent front. In this environment, asking for help can feel like failure.

But the truth is, seeking support is not a sign of weakness. It's an act of strength. It takes courage to say, "I'm not okay," and even more to take steps toward healing. As healthcare professionals, we need to start modelling this courage for each other. Recovery is not a solo journey — it requires a shift in our collective mindset. We need to actively foster workplaces where vulnerability is not only accepted but supported. Where taking a mental health day is seen as just as valid as treating a physical illness. Where someone stepping back for their well-being is respected, not judged.

Thriving in healthcare shouldn't come at the cost of our humanity. The well-being of those providing care must be valued just as highly as the care itself. Because when we're supported — emotionally, mentally, and structurally — we're able to show up as our best selves. Not just for our patients, but for each other, our families, and most importantly, ourselves.

Chapter 5

Emotionally Intelligent Leadership and Team Culture

5.1 Leading Yourself First: The Heart of Emotionally Intelligent Leadership

"Mastering others is strength; mastering oneself is true power."

— Lao Tsu

EMOTIONALLY INTELLIGENT LEADERSHIP TRAITS

It's important to understand that leadership isn't reserved for those in formal positions of authority. As John C. Maxwell puts it, "*Everyone is a leader because everyone influences someone.*" Whether through our actions, our words, or simply by the example we set, we all carry the potential to lead.

In successful organisations, leadership is everyone's responsibility. It's not about hierarchy — it's about taking initiative, lifting others up, and contributing to a shared vision. When we adopt this mindset, we create teams where leadership is distributed, all voices are heard, and everyone feels empowered to make a meaningful impact.

Emotionally intelligent leadership starts from within. Before we can truly lead others — before we inspire, guide, or support — we must learn to know and lead ourselves. That means understanding our emotions, motivations, and the role we play in the energy and direction of our team.

This process begins with self-awareness which is the foundation of all emotionally intelligent leadership. We need to be able to recognise what we're feeling in the moment and how those feelings might be influencing our behaviour. For example, if I'm feeling frustrated, I try to pause and ask myself: "Where is this coming from?" and "Is this the right moment to speak?" It's about creating that space between feeling and reacting as we have discussed so often already — so that we respond with intention, not emotion. That kind of pause doesn't just protect team morale, it builds it.

Next comes self-motivation. This is the internal drive that keeps us moving forward, especially on the tough days. And in healthcare, we all know there are tough days. This isn't just about ticking boxes or reaching external goals — it's about showing up because we care. It's the kind of motivation that comes from knowing our *why*. For me, it's the people — my patients, my team, my family. That inner compass helps us stay grounded and keep perspective, even when the pressure is on.

Self-accountability is just as critical. Leaders don't just own their wins — they take responsibility when things don't go to plan. It's not always easy to say, "I got that wrong," but when we do, we create a culture where honesty, trust, and learning are the norm. Accountability, when modelled well, helps everyone feel safe enough to own their mistakes and grow from them, instead of hiding them out of fear.

Adaptability is another vital trait — especially in healthcare, where unpredictability is part of the job. Emotionally intelligent leaders can pivot quickly without losing their footing. They stay open to new information, adjust strategies when needed, and remain calm in the face of uncertainty. This doesn't mean having all the answers — it means being able to lead with flexibility and composure when plans change. And just as importantly, they communicate those changes clearly, helping their teams feel supported and steady even when the path ahead is shifting.

Then there's empathy — the ability to really tune in to how others are feeling and show them that they're seen and supported. In healthcare, this is everything. When we lead with empathy, we don't just tell people what to do — we listen, we validate, and we respond in ways that build connection. Especially during stressful or uncertain moments, empathetic leadership helps teams stay calm, cohesive, and focused on what matters most.

In the end, emotionally intelligent leaders lead by example. They create workplaces where people feel respected, heard, and encouraged to be their best selves. They model vulnerability, self-reflection, and accountability — and in doing so, invite others to do the same.

Reflection: Leading from Within

Take a quiet moment — before or after a busy day — and sit somewhere you won't be interrupted. Bring a journal, notes app, or even just a few sticky notes. This is about checking in with yourself, honestly and without judgment. Ask yourself the following questions:

1. Self-Awareness

- *What emotion showed up most often for me at work this week — frustration, stress, joy, excitement, something else?*
- *How did that emotion shape the way I showed up as a leader or teammate?*
- *Was there a moment where I reacted instead of responded? What might I do differently next time?*

2. *Self-Motivation*

- *Why do I show up to lead?*
- *What's one thing that re-centres me when I'm losing focus or feeling overwhelmed?*
- *Did I model the kind of energy and attitude I want to see in my team this week?*

3. *Self-Accountability*

- *Where did I do well this week — and where did I fall short?*
- *Did I take ownership for both outcomes and behaviours, even when things didn't go to plan?*
- *What's one conversation I've been avoiding that I need to have?*

4. *Empathy*

- *When was the last time I asked someone on my team how they're really doing?*
- *Did I create space for someone to share openly — or was I too busy to notice?*
- *How did I respond to someone else's stress or emotion today? Was it with patience and presence?*

5. *Action Step*

- *Based on these reflections, what's one small thing I'll do differently tomorrow to show up as a more emotionally intelligent leader?*

This doesn't have to be a long process — even 10 minutes of reflection can give you significant insight and clarity. Try returning to this once a week or after particularly challenging leadership moments. Over time, you'll notice patterns — and the better you know yourself, the better equipped you'll be to support those around you.

REAL STORIES OF EMOTIONALLY INTELLIGENT LEADERSHIP IN ACTION

Emotionally intelligent leadership isn't just a nice idea — it changes lives. It shows up in real clinical environments and creates ripple effects you can feel in both team culture and patient outcomes. I want to share two stories from a local hospital that highlight just how powerful this kind of leadership can be in healthcare settings.

Let's start with a paediatric ward in a public hospital that was facing a string of challenges — high staff turnover, rising patient complaints, and a general sense of burnout across the board. The nursing team was struggling, with many feeling unsupported and unheard, especially during busy shifts when patient load was high. Then, a new head nurse came on board. She didn't arrive guns blazing with a new policy manual; instead, she led with empathy and curiosity. Her first move was to sit down with every single member of the team and just listen. She asked questions like, "What's making your day harder than it needs to be?" and "What would help you feel more supported at work?"

In these enquiry sessions, it became clear that one of the biggest issues wasn't necessarily the workload itself — it was the way it was being distributed. Some nurses were regularly staying back late while others were finishing early. Others were struggling with a lack of mentorship and felt like they were constantly in survival mode without adequate support from senior staff. So, the head nurse began making subtle but powerful changes — adjusting shift pairings to provide better support, introducing informal peer check-ins at the start of each day, and celebrating small wins more consistently. Slowly but surely, morale began to shift. Nurses began sticking around, offering to cover shifts for one another, and patient satisfaction scores started to climb. The culture turned from one of burnout to one of belonging.

Another powerful example comes from a surgical department where communication breakdowns had led to near-miss incidents. There was a culture of silence — junior staff were hesitant to speak up when they noticed problems, especially if a senior surgeon was involved. This kind of environment is unfortunately all too common. One survey found that while 84% of healthcare professionals had seen colleagues take potentially unsafe shortcuts, less than half felt safe enough to speak up about it. That's a dangerous space to be operating in — literally.

In this department, a senior surgeon decided to break the cycle. He noticed the pattern and instead of blaming the team, he created a new system of regular pre- and post-op debriefs. But it wasn't just a checklist — it was about culture. He made a point of going last in every roundtable discussion, so everyone else had a chance to speak freely. He normalised questions and welcomed even the most hesitant feedback by responding with curiosity rather than criticism. He'd say things like, "Tell me more about that," or "Thanks for noticing — what do you think we can do differently next time?"

He also made it a point to call out positive behaviour publicly — when a junior doctor flagged a minor discrepancy in a patient's chart before surgery, he stopped the team mid-discussion to thank them and explain why it mattered. That's the kind of moment that changes culture. Soon enough, it wasn't just the junior doctors speaking up. Nurses, anaesthetists, even admin staff began flagging concerns early, which led to fewer errors and a huge improvement in team cohesion.

The transformation didn't happen overnight, but it was powerful. Not only were there fewer safety incidents, but the team itself became tighter. They trusted each other. They knew they could speak up, that their voice mattered, and that it would be received with respect. For trainees, this kind of psychological safety is essential. It allows them to engage, ask questions, and admit when they don't know something — without fear of judgement. And when you create that kind of space, everyone benefits, especially the patients.

These stories show us what emotionally intelligent leadership really looks like in practice. It's not about grand gestures or rigid policies — it's about being present, listening, and creating an environment where people feel seen and safe. It's about setting the tone for a culture where people take ownership, support each other, and feel empowered to do their best work. That's when the magic happens — when care becomes collaborative, and leadership becomes something that lives at every level of the organisation.

STRATEGIES TO DEVELOP YOUR LEADERSHIP SKILLS

If you're aiming to grow as a leader in healthcare, it starts with a good, honest look inward. Leadership isn't about having all the answers — it's about understanding yourself well enough to guide others with authenticity, compassion, and clarity. That's the foundation of emotional intelligence. Developing this kind of leadership style means tuning in to your own emotional responses and how they impact those around you. It requires ongoing reflection, a willingness to grow, and the courage to ask, "How can I do better?"

A great place to start is by evaluating your own strengths and growth areas when it comes to emotional intelligence. Are you aware of how you come across under stress? Can you stay calm and composed when things go off-script? How comfortable are you with giving — and receiving — feedback? Tools like the EQ-i 2.0 or Emotional Intelligence Appraisal can be really helpful here. They give you a structured way to assess things like self-awareness, empathy, and social skills, helping you get clear on where you already shine and where there's room to grow. But don't feel you need a formal test to begin — you can also do this by reflecting on past experiences and asking trusted colleagues for honest input.

One of the best habits I've built into my own routine is mindfulness. Just a few minutes each day — either during a quiet moment before clinic or in the car before I head in — helps me check in with how I'm feeling. Am I carrying stress from home into work? Is something already making me feel irritable or rushed? Being able to pause, notice, and reset has helped me respond rather than react. That kind of emotional regulation isn't just about staying calm — it helps you be more present with patients, more grounded with your team, and more in control when the pressure is on. Mindfulness doesn't need to look like sitting on a cushion with your eyes closed; it could be a quiet moment walking your dog or simply taking three deep breaths before a difficult conversation.

Another powerful tool is feedback. I know it can feel uncomfortable at times, but getting honest input from your team is one of the fastest ways to grow as a leader. Ask people you trust, "How do you experience me when I'm under pressure?" or "Is there anything I could be doing differently to support the team better?" Sometimes, you'll find that a habit you thought was helpful — like jumping in to fix things quickly — might actually be undermining someone's confidence.

A few years ago, we had a relatively new team member resign not long after starting. At the time, we were going through major staff turnover, and the culture hadn't quite settled. In her resignation email, she shared that a key reason for leaving was that "the suction and other dental tools were snatched from my hands forcefully in front of patients," which she felt undermined her and created a poor learning environment. In dentistry, especially when working with someone new, it's common to step in and take the suction to prevent contamination or make the patient more comfortable — particularly when the assistant can't fully see into the mouth. It's often done automatically, without speaking, to keep things seamless for the patient. But in this case, it clearly came across very differently to her. Looking back, I realised she probably didn't feel safe enough to raise her concerns earlier — or maybe I just didn't check in soon enough to invite that conversation. Either way, it was a missed opportunity for mutual understanding and growth.

That experience really stuck with me. Feedback — especially when it's early and honest — can prevent these kinds of misunderstandings from escalating. It gives you a chance to adjust with intention, rather than continuing patterns that don't serve you or your team.

Role-playing scenarios can also be incredibly useful for building empathy and sharpening your leadership instincts. You might practise how to respond when a team member is underperforming, or what to say when a junior clinician expresses doubt about a treatment decision. These aren't just theoretical exercises — they're opportunities to practice compassion in real time and prepare for the moments that matter most. For example, imagine a young nurse pulling you aside to share a concern about a colleague who's cutting corners during procedures. How you respond — whether you create safety or shut them down — has a massive impact. Practising these conversations helps you lead with empathy and create a culture where people feel heard.

Empathy-building doesn't stop there. Another simple but powerful practice is reflective listening. When a team member opens up about a challenge, try summarising what you've heard before offering advice. For example, if a team member says they're feeling overwhelmed with the new booking system, instead of jumping in with a fix, you might say, "It sounds like the changes have made your day feel a lot more chaotic — have I got that right?" This signals that you're not just hearing them — you're trying to understand. That kind of connection can make people feel supported and safe to speak up.

Asking clarifying or reflective questions not only helps ensure you've understood the real issue — it can also be an opportunity to empower the team member to find their own solution. Again, instead of immediately offering a fix, you might ask, "What do you think would help make it feel more manageable?" or "Have you noticed any parts of the system that are working well so far?" These kinds of questions invite them to think critically, build confidence, and strengthen their own leadership instincts. Over time, this approach helps create a team that doesn't just rely on you for answers — they start seeing themselves as problem solvers too.

It's also worth paying attention to the emotional cues your team is giving you. Are people withdrawing from conversations? Getting snappy or defensive in situations where they'd normally be composed? Showing up late, looking tired, or simply not bringing the same energy they once did? These behaviours often signal that something deeper is going on — stress, overwhelm, or even early signs of burnout. Leaders with high emotional intelligence don't ignore these cues. They notice, they care, and most importantly, they act.

Checking in doesn't need to be a formal process. Sometimes it's as simple as taking someone aside and saying, "You've seemed a bit flat this week — is everything okay?" or "I've noticed you haven't been yourself lately, and I just wanted to check in." These small, human moments communicate that you see your team not just as workers, but as people. And when done genuinely and without judgment, they can open the door for honest conversation and early support.

Even if the team member doesn't share much in that moment, your check-in still plants a seed — it signals that their wellbeing matters, and that if and when they're ready to talk, you'll be there. Over time, these micro-moments of care build something powerful: trust. And with trust comes psychological safety — the foundation of every high-performing, connected team.

And of course, never underestimate the value of ongoing learning. I've found that reading, listening to podcasts, and attending leadership workshops keeps me inspired and helps me bring fresh ideas to my practice. Books like *Emotional Intelligence 2.0* by Dr. Travis Bradberry and *Dare to Lead* by Brené Brown have been favourites of mine. They're filled with practical strategies that are easy to implement, even in a busy clinical setting. And sometimes, just hearing how other leaders have navigated similar challenges is enough to spark a breakthrough of your own.

THE EQ LEADERSHIP FRAMEWORK

I'm a big believer in having something visual to guide the process — especially when it comes to emotional intelligence, which can sometimes feel a bit abstract. That's why I've created a simplified visual framework to map out the key elements of emotionally intelligent leadership in healthcare. It serves as a high-level snapshot — a reminder of how self-awareness, regulation, motivation, empathy, communication, and culture all connect to create meaningful impact.

Each element in the framework links to deeper, practical and actionable strategies. Because this isn't just about theory — it's about real-world leadership. EQ isn't something we master once and tick off a list: it's something we practise, refine, and build over time. It's a lifelong journey of learning, growing, and evolving as both a clinician and a leader. My hope is that this framework helps keep that journey grounded — serving as both a practical tool and a visual reminder that leading with heart isn't just possible, it's powerful.

Let's walk through the roadmap for applying emotional intelligence in healthcare leadership together — step by step:

1. Self-Awareness (Start Here)

"I know myself."

- Reflect daily: What did I do well? What could I do better?
- Use journaling to track emotional triggers and recurring patterns.
- Complete a formal EQ self-assessment (e.g. EQ-i 2.0, ESCI).

- Ask for honest feedback from trusted team members or mentors.

Leads to...

2. Self-Regulation

"I manage myself well under pressure."

- Practice mindfulness, breathing techniques or progressive muscle relaxation (PMR).
- Use techniques like emotional labelling and emotional distancing.
- Identify early signs of stress or burnout and take proactive steps.
- Pause before responding — especially in emotionally charged situations.

Leads to...

3. Motivation

"I stay driven by purpose."

- Reconnect with your personal "why" during high-pressure times.
- Set meaningful, values-aligned goals — personally and for your team.
- Celebrate progress and small wins to maintain momentum.
- Stay committed to the bigger picture, even when challenges arise.

Leads to...

4. Empathy

"I understand and value what others feel."

- Practice reflective listening during patient and team conversations.
- Use perspective-taking to better understand your team's point of view.
- Check in regularly: "How are you doing? What can I do to support you?"
- Use shared language, analogies, or visual aids to help patients and team members feel seen and understood.

Leads to...

5. Social Skills & Team Dynamics

"I help others thrive."

- Set clear expectations and communicate with kindness and clarity.
- Hold regular debriefs, check-ins, and huddles to improve connection.
- Acknowledge personal milestones and wins — professionally and personally.
- Give feedback with empathy, receive feedback with grace and openness.

Leads to...

6. Service-Driven Leadership

"I lead by lifting others."

- Empower team members to lead from where they are.
- Celebrate contributions and give credit where it's due.
- Be willing to roll up your sleeves — no task is beneath you.

- Focus on shared purpose: connect everything back to the mission and vision.

Leads to...

7. The Ripple Effect

"Leadership becomes cultural, not positional."

- Team feels heard, supported, and empowered.
- Psychological safety increases — people speak up, innovate, and grow.
- Patient care improves because team connection is stronger.
- Resilience, retention, and trust all grow organically.

EQ LEADERSHIP FRAMEWORK

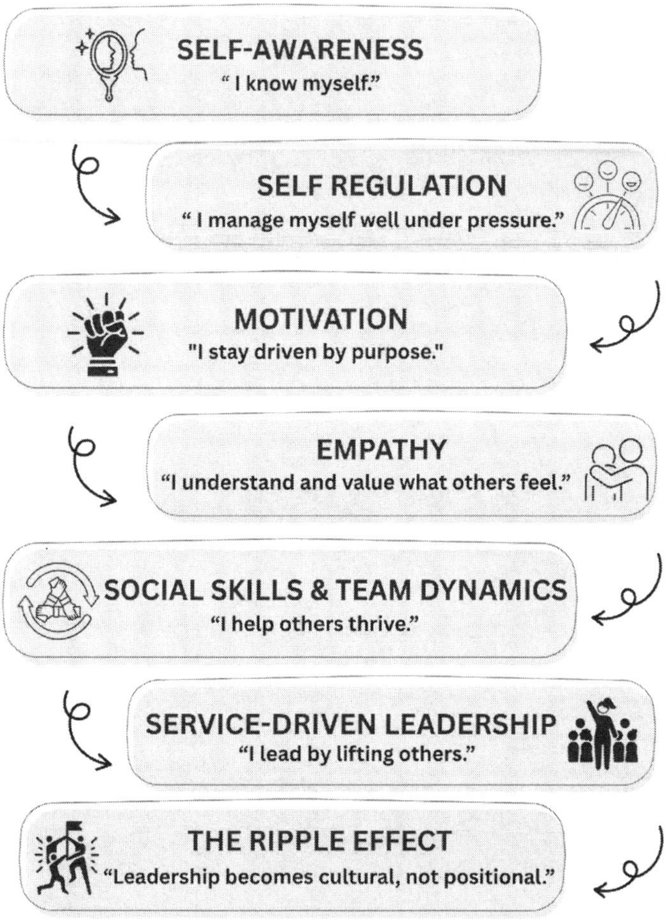

5.2 The Listening Shift: Transforming Teams through Active Listening

---

"Most of the successful people I've known are the ones who do more listening than talking."

— Bernard M. Baruch

As we've discussed, active listening is one of the most underrated yet powerful skills we need to master — and one that often gets overshadowed by the fast pace and problem-solving mindset of clinical environments. If we want to build high-functioning teams and deliver truly excellent care, creating a culture of listening isn't just helpful — it's foundational.

WHY LISTENING IS FOUNDATIONAL TO LEADERSHIP

Active listening means being fully present — not just hearing the words, but tuning in to the tone, the body language, and the emotion behind the words. It's about curiosity rather than assumption, connection over correction. And it starts with us. It is an act of humility – recognising that understanding comes from being open to others' perspectives, not simply voicing our own. When we choose to pause our own agenda and truly listen, we model the kind of respect and openness that builds trust, collaboration and psychological safety — three non-negotiables in any healthcare team.

One of the most powerful tools we can use to practise this is reflective listening. That's when we paraphrase or repeat key parts of what someone has said to confirm our understanding. It might sound simple, but it's incredibly effective. For example, if a team member says, "I just feel like I can't catch up lately — everything's piling on," you might respond, "It sounds like you're feeling stretched really thin at the moment. Is that right?" Or if someone says, "I'm not sure if I handled that patient call the right way," you could reply, "It sounds like you're second-guessing how it went and want to make sure you did the right thing. Would it help to talk it through together?" These small, intentional moments of reflection send a powerful message: I hear you, and I care about what you're saying. In doing so, we don't just confirm understanding — we demonstrate care, respect, and a willingness to collaborate. We're not just confirming accuracy — we're affirming respect, trust, and a willingness to support.

FROM COMPLIANCE TO CONTRIBUTION

Open-ended questions are another key to creating meaningful dialogue. They shift the focus from passive agreement to active contribution. Instead of asking close-ended questions like "Do you agree?" or "Is that okay?", try asking, "How do you feel about this plan?", "What do you think we might be missing?", or "What would make this feel more workable for you?" These types of questions open the door to new perspectives and signal that you genuinely value the other person's insight. They also help uncover hidden concerns or ideas that might otherwise go unspoken. In team settings, this shifts the dynamic from hierarchical to collaborative — from top-down to side-by-side. That's exactly the kind of relational strength we need in high-pressure, high-stakes environments like healthcare, where psychological safety is essential for both team wellbeing and patient care.

LISTENING IS A SAFETY PRACTICE

The impact of active listening can't be overstated. Miscommunication is one of the most common contributors to medical errors, fractured team dynamics, and poor patient outcomes. In high-pressure environments, even a single misunderstood instruction or unchecked assumption can set off a chain reaction. A rushed comment, a vague handover, or a missed emotional cue — these moments may seem small but carry serious weight.

When we take time to truly listen — reflecting, clarifying, and staying present — we dramatically reduce those risks. It's not about slowing down clinical work — it's about being intentional with our attention. That small shift in how we show up has a big impact: clearer communication, stronger collaboration, and a safer environment for both patients and teams. Listening isn't just a soft skill — it's a leadership strength, a safety measure, and a cultural anchor.

FROM SKILL TO CULTURE: WHEN LISTENING TRANSFORMS TEAMS

I'll never forget a story a physician friend of mine shared with me. He was working in a busy tertiary hospital where his department had been struggling with burnout, poor communication, and frequent friction between junior and senior staff. People were walking on eggshells. Patient handovers felt more like ticking boxes than genuine exchanges.

The turning point came when a new head of department noticed the tension and made an unexpected shift. Instead of focusing the next meeting on metrics or procedures, he asked everyone to share what was most challenging in their workday. No interruptions — just listening. What started as awkward silence turned into a cascade of stories: nurses overwhelmed by unacknowledged workloads, junior doctors afraid to ask for help, admin staff feeling invisible.

That one act of listening cracked something open. In the weeks that followed, they introduced small but consistent listening practices — team check-ins, reflective summaries during rounds, and a renewed focus on open dialogue. Gradually, trust grew. Communication became clearer, conflicts decreased, and — most importantly — patient outcomes improved.

This story stays with me because it shows what happens when leaders treat listening as a priority, not a nicety. Listening is not passive. It's a conscious, active choice that can shift culture from the inside out. It doesn't require a new policy manual — just presence, empathy, and consistency. As healthcare leaders — regardless of our job title — we have the power and responsibility to shape culture through how we show up. When we lead with genuine presence and empathy, we model what safe, respectful communication looks like.

When listening becomes the norm, not the exception, something shifts: people speak up, ideas flow, morale lifts, and patient care improves. It all starts with hearing — not just what's said, but what's really meant.

5.3 Emotional Awareness in Action: What Makes Teams Thrive

> *"When dealing with people, remember you are not dealing with creatures of logic, but with creatures of emotion."*
>
> — Dale Carnegie

At the heart of a truly cohesive, high-performing team is emotional awareness. Not just awareness of our own emotions, but of those around us — the subtle signals, the unspoken tensions, and the emotional "climate" of the room. We can't leave our feelings at the door when we walk into a healthcare environment, nor should we. Every team member brings not only their clinical skills and knowledge, but also their emotional experiences — the highs, the frustrations, the personal pressures — that influence how they show up at work. The way we navigate these emotions as a team is what sets a functional group apart from a truly supportive, collaborative one.

When we acknowledge and create space for emotions at work — especially after high-stress situations or new challenges — we help prevent burnout, reduce conflict, and foster connection. That doesn't mean we need to turn every team meeting into a therapy session — but it *does* mean recognising when someone needs space to unpack something, or when a debrief could help prevent emotions from simmering under the surface.

One of the best ways to encourage this is through group reflections. These don't have to be formal or time-consuming. Sometimes, they're just a quick check-in after a difficult patient interaction or a new experience — an opportunity to say, "That was a lot. How are you feeling about it?"

DEBRIEFING WITH HEART: TURNING CHALLENGES INTO CONNECTION

Just recently, one of my new associates — a lovely new grad — did her very first crown on a patient. The appointment went well overall, but as expected, there were a few hiccups and moments that could have been smoother. After the appointment, she, the dental assistant, and I sat down for a debrief — not to critique her performance, but to support her as she processed the experience. She was able to articulate how she felt — nervous, ashamed, relieved, even a little overwhelmed — and that opened the door for us to talk through those emotions together. I gave her feedback on the technical aspects, yes, but more importantly, I helped her reframe the situation as a learning experience and importantly, as a win overall. Not because it was perfect, but because she faced her fear and did it. The assistant chimed in too — not with criticism, but with gentle observations about her communication with the patient during the appointment, helping her see how she came across in the room. It was such a powerful moment of shared support and emotional unpacking — and a great reminder that it's not just what we reflect on that matters, but how we hold space for one another in those vulnerable moments.

Moments like this are rare in busy clinical settings. We're often so focused on productivity, efficiency, and outcomes that we forget to create space for emotional reflection — especially for new graduates still finding their feet. But it's in these quiet, honest conversations that the most meaningful learning and growth can happen. Taking time for emotional debriefs is a leadership practice that builds safety, confidence, and trust.

STRENGTHENING EMOTIONAL AWARENESS IN TEAMS

There are plenty of simple yet impactful ways to develop emotional awareness within a team — starting with creating moments of reflection and shared understanding. Group reflections, like the one shared earlier, are a powerful place to start. They normalise emotional processing as part of clinical practice, helping team members feel seen and supported rather than judged. Even short, informal check-ins after a challenging case — "That was a tough one. How are you feeling?" — can open up space for validation, connection, and deeper learning.

Another effective tool is role-reversal exercises. These don't need to be dramatic or theatrical — just taking a moment to imagine someone else's experience can be eye-opening. For instance, asking a dentist to picture a day in the life of a dental assistant — juggling sterilisation, managing nervous patients, resetting rooms, and anticipating clinician needs at the same time — can dramatically shift the way they communicate and delegate. The reverse is also true: helping dental assistants understand the mental load of clinical decision-making and time pressures can spark mutual respect. This mutual empathy builds stronger, more collaborative relationships.

Workshops focused on emotional intelligence, team dynamics, or burnout prevention can also create opportunities for shared learning and vulnerability. These sessions don't just teach tools — they open conversations. When team members hear each other describe similar emotional challenges, it fosters connection and reduces the isolation that often creeps in during high-stress periods.

One activity I particularly love is emotional mapping. This involves tracking your emotions at key points throughout the workday and then reflecting on those patterns as a group. For example: "When do I feel the most supported?" "When do I notice my energy dip?" "What situations consistently leave me feeling stressed or deflated?" These patterns reveal emotional hotspots — places where support systems can be strengthened or small changes can make a big difference.

Even visual tools like colour-coded mood boards, anonymous pulse surveys, or sticky-note feedback walls can help foster a culture of emotional honesty — especially in teams that are still developing trust. The key isn't perfection — it's consistency and care. When leaders create regular, safe spaces to reflect and share emotional experiences, it sends a powerful message: that how people feel at work matters, and that emotional awareness is a strength, not a weakness.

READING THE EMOTIONAL ROOM

While structured reflections and shared activities help strengthen emotional awareness as a team, leaders also need to develop a more instinctive ability to tune into the emotional tone of the room day-to-day. This is because leaders play a crucial role in shaping and safeguarding the emotional health of a team — and it often begins with what isn't said. Reading the emotional room means tuning into the subtle shifts in energy, behaviour, and atmosphere that can signal underlying stress, tension, or disengagement. It's a form of emotional radar, and emotionally intelligent leaders know how to use it.

Maybe a normally chatty team member has gone unusually quiet. Maybe your usually upbeat assistant seems irritable or flat. Maybe the whole team feels heavier than usual — less laughter, more eye-rolls, longer silences. These may seem like small moments, but they're rarely random. More often than not, they're signs of something deeper: burnout creeping in, an unresolved conflict, or someone struggling silently.

Paying attention to these cues doesn't require a special title — it just takes presence. It's about noticing patterns, not just events. A single off day might be nothing. But a gradual change in someone's mood, tone, or behaviour is worth exploring.

One-on-one check-ins are one of the most powerful tools here. These don't have to be formal. A simple, "You seem a bit off this week — want to talk about anything?" can open the door. The key is to approach it with curiosity, not judgment. The goal isn't to fix everything on the spot, but to show that you care and that you're paying attention.

You can also make emotional health part of your team's shared language. Short, anonymous pulse surveys (e.g. "How are you feeling about work this week — from energised to exhausted?") or colour-coded check-ins at team huddles ("Red, yellow, green — how's everyone feeling today?") can normalise emotional expression without requiring people to be overly vulnerable. Over time, this helps create a psychologically safe culture where emotions are acknowledged rather than suppressed.

And here's the ripple effect: when leaders show they're attuned to the emotional undercurrents of the workplace, it gives everyone else permission to do the same. People begin checking in on each other, communicating earlier, and creating a culture of mutual care rather than silent struggle.

Because ultimately, reading the room is about more than observation — it's about action. It's the choice to pause, notice, and respond with intention. And when you do that consistently, you become the kind of leader people feel safe around — not just professionally, but personally too.

HEALTHY BOUNDARIES STRENGTHEN TREAMS

Of course, acknowledging emotion doesn't mean carrying every team member's emotional load or becoming overly entangled in their experiences. We also need boundaries — clear ones. Healthy boundaries are what allow vulnerability to exist without leading to burnout. They create the psychological "guardrails" that let us be present and compassionate without becoming overwhelmed or depleted. When teams have strong boundaries, they're actually more able — not less — to connect, collaborate, and support one another safely.

Boundaries aren't about shutting feelings down. They're about creating structure and shared expectations so we can all express ourselves honestly and sustainably. They offer clarity around what's okay, what's not, and what's needed for emotional safety. For example, daily check-ins and end-of-day "check-outs" can create a rhythm for emotional expression — without expecting people to be available at all times. They also normalise emotional fluctuations, giving people language and space to say "I'm not okay today" without stigma.

One powerful way to reinforce team boundaries is by creating a team charter — a short, collaboratively built document that outlines how the team agrees to communicate, handle conflict, and support each other. It might include agreements like:

- "We speak respectfully, even when frustrated."
- "We don't gossip."
- "We ask before venting."
- "We assume positive intent."
- "We make space for honest feedback — and receive it with grace and openness."

These kinds of shared norms are especially valuable during onboarding, high-stress periods, or cultural shifts. They remove ambiguity and empower everyone to uphold a respectful and emotionally safe workplace. And importantly, when boundaries are honoured consistently by leadership, they set the tone for the rest of the team — showing that wellbeing is not just talked about but actively protected.

Because ultimately, boundaries aren't barriers — they're bridges to better communication, stronger trust, and more sustainable connection.

5.4 Creating a Culture of Open Communication and Psychological Safety

---

"Sensitivity to others is no trivial skill; rather, it is a truly precious human ability. But it isn't complex: it requires receptiveness to other people and a willingness to listen."

— James Kouzes and Barry Posner

PRINCIPLES OF OPEN COMMUNICATION

Building a culture of open communication starts with a commitment to honesty, clarity, and inclusivity. It means creating a space where every team member — from the most senior specialist to the newest trainee — feels safe, heard, and valued. For instance, when a junior assistant feels safe enough to speak up about an instrument tray they're unsure about, it might prevent a serious procedural delay or error. Open communication isn't about who talks the most or who has the final say — it's about encouraging contribution, collaboration, and curiosity at every level.

Honesty builds trust. Whether we're discussing treatment plans for patients, giving feedback, or raising concerns, being honest (while still being kind) is what allows relationships to flourish and decisions to be made with confidence. Clarity ensures our messages don't get lost in translation. We all know how easily things can be misunderstood in a fast-paced environment like healthcare — so taking the extra moment to be clear, to confirm understanding, is always worth it. And inclusivity means more than just welcoming different opinions — it's about actively seeking out and valuing them, knowing that the best ideas often come from the most unexpected places.

In my experience, the best teams thrive when they know that every role matters. It's something I feel strongly about — no one is more important than anyone else. The person cleaning the surgery at the end of the day is just as vital to safe, effective patient care as the clinician in the chair. Everyone contributes. When we make space for every voice and treat every contribution with respect, we create a team that's not only more connected — but far more effective.

EMOTIONALLY INTELLIGENT COMMUNICATION TECHNIQUES

Emotionally intelligent communication is about so much more than just exchanging information — it's about connection, clarity, and trust. It's how we make others feel heard, valued, and safe enough to open up. One of the most powerful techniques is empathetic mirroring — reflecting back not just the words, but the emotion behind what someone is saying. For example, if a team member is clearly overwhelmed after a tough shift, something as simple as, "It sounds like today really took it out of you," can go a long way in validating how they feel. When we feel truly heard, something shifts — there's a release of the emotional pressure we've been carrying, and in that space, our minds begin to settle, which actually opens up our ability to problem-solve.

Another simple but underutilised technique is the pause. In emotionally charged or sensitive conversations, allowing space for silence gives everyone a moment to reflect and respond more thoughtfully rather than reactively. It's a small gesture that fosters deeper, more respectful dialogue — and it signals that you're genuinely present and listening.

We also talk a lot in our clinic about solution-oriented language. It's not about ignoring problems or sugar-coating reality — it's about how we frame challenges in a way that keeps the conversation constructive. For example, instead of saying, "You keep forgetting to update the patient notes," a more productive approach might be, "How can we make it easier to stay on top of patient notes going forward?" It shifts the tone from blame to collaboration and sends a clear message: we're here to work through this together.

Another tool we actively use in my practice is the Above vs Below the Line model shown below — a framework that helps us recognise whether our thinking and behaviour are coming from a place of curiosity, responsibility, and openness (above the line), or from defensiveness, blame, and closed-mindedness (below the line). For example, above the line might sound like, "Let's figure this out together," while below the line might be, "That's not my problem."

We've got a copy of this image up on the whiteboard in the clinic, and every new team member is introduced to it as part of their onboarding. We refer to it all the time — during debriefs, check-ins, or even just as gentle reminders throughout the day. It helps us hold ourselves and each other accountable in a way that feels respectful and grounded. Fostering this kind of mindset is one of the most powerful ways to build a culture where open, honest, emotionally intelligent communication becomes the norm — not the exception. When we use these techniques consistently, we create a workplace where communication isn't just about efficiency — it's about building connection, trust, and a shared commitment to doing our best work, together.

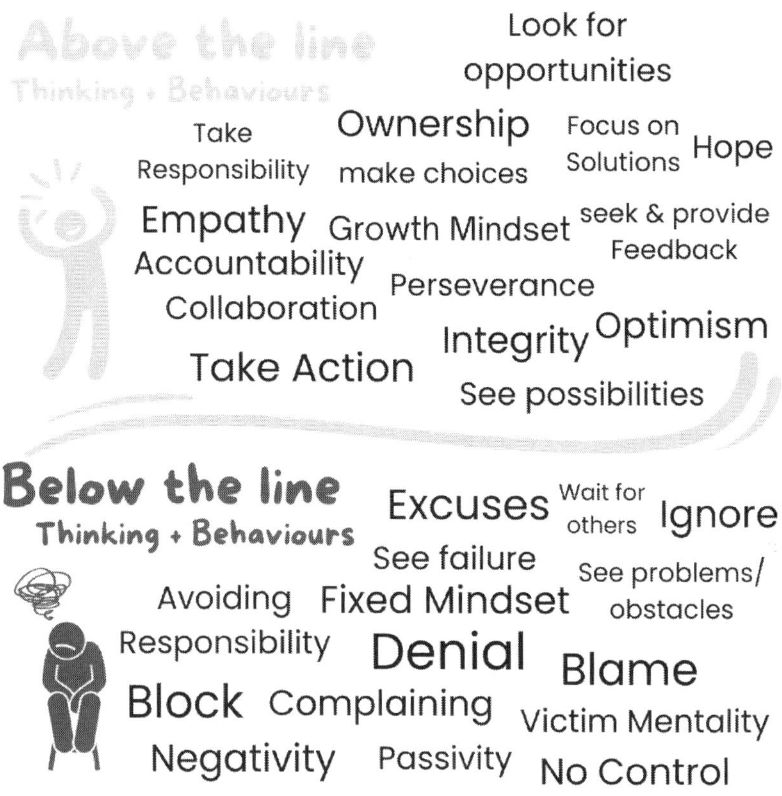

CREATING SAFE SPACES FOR DIALOGUE

If we want our teams to thrive — not just function — we have to create spaces where people feel safe to speak up. Safe spaces, both physical and emotional, are essential in building a culture of trust and openness. These are the environments where people feel they can share concerns, frustrations, or even new ideas without fear of being dismissed, judged, or facing repercussions. And leaders need these spaces too — safe, peer-level conversations help prevent isolation and burnout.

In practical terms, this could look like a quiet office for one-on-one conversations, a scheduled team huddle where everyone has the opportunity to share, or even a casual chat in the staff room. It's less about the location and more about the atmosphere. These spaces become a container for honesty and connection — and when used intentionally, they can transform team morale, cohesion, and effectiveness. This applies to leaders just as much as anyone else on the team.

But safe spaces don't magically appear. They're built — intentionally, day by day — through the culture we create. And culture is not defined by a poster on the wall or a line in a mission statement. It's what happens in the micro-moments: how we speak to each other under pressure, how we handle feedback, how safe it feels to ask a question, share an idea, or say, "I'm not okay."

In my practice, I try to reinforce this daily. I make it a habit to check in with my team — not just on the logistics of the day, but on how they're doing as people. "Are you okay? Is there anything I can do to support you?" It's a small question, but it often opens the door to bigger conversations. And these moments aren't just about putting out fires — they're about sending a clear message: You matter here.

THE STRENGTH IN VULNERABILITY

A critical ingredient in creating safe spaces is vulnerability. And as much as we might want to avoid it, vulnerability is not a weakness — it's the cornerstone of psychological safety and a key driver of authentic relationships. When we as leaders are willing to be human — to admit when something's hard, when we've made a mistake, or when we don't have all the answers — we give others permission to do the same. That openness builds trust faster than any team-building exercise ever could.

That doesn't mean spilling your guts or sharing every personal detail. Vulnerability is about thoughtful honesty and being intentionally open. If I'm feeling the weight of a particularly stressful or demanding appointment, I might say, "I found that appointment really tough today — how did you go?" or "This week's been full on.

Is anyone else feeling it?" It's these kinds of genuine, grounded check-ins that create space for others to open up too.

In fact, I remember a day not long ago where things were particularly hectic. Instead of powering through and pretending everything was fine, I said to the team, "I'm feeling pretty stretched today – how's everyone else travelling?" The shift in the room was immediate. One of the team members shared something that had been bothering her, and we ended up having a really productive conversation that might never have happened otherwise. That's the power of vulnerability – it sets the tone for honest, supportive dialogue.

But here's the thing: vulnerability doesn't work in isolation and is not always easy to embrace. It needs to be supported by a culture that honours it. Many of us fear rejection or judgment when we expose our true selves, particularly in professional settings. There's often an underlying anxiety: "What if people think less of me if they know how I'm really feeling?" For us as healthcare professionals, who are often expected to project strength and competence, this fear can be magnified. Yet, the benefits of vulnerability far outweigh these fears. By being open, we dismantle the culture of invalidation that can pervade workplaces, where people feel they are only as good as their last mistake. Vulnerability helps create an environment where every team member feels valued and understood, reducing anxiety and unpredictability in interpersonal dynamics.

THE IMPACT OF MUTUAL RESPECT

Respect isn't just a courtesy; it's a cornerstone of effective teamwork. Respect also isn't passive – it's shown in how we acknowledge each other's work, say thank you, and give credit where it's due. In my view, respect is a two-way street: you have to give respect to get it. No one in the team is more important than anyone else, and everyone deserves to feel valued for their contributions.

When team members feel respected, they're more engaged, motivated, and willing to go the extra mile. Respect shows up in small but meaningful ways — listening attentively, considering each other's ideas, and treating everyone with dignity, regardless of their role. These actions create a positive workplace culture where people want to stay, reducing turnover and improving team morale.

This mutual respect then naturally extends to patient care. Teams that respect each other are more cohesive and collaborative, which translates into better communication and more personalised, empathetic care. Patients feel this difference — they sense when they're in an environment where every team member is aligned in their commitment to providing the best possible care. It builds trust, fosters compliance, and ultimately leads to better outcomes by elevating the standard of care we deliver every day.

5.5 Trust in Action: The Heart of a High-Performing Team

"Trust is the foundation of leadership."

— Colin Powell

TRUST: THE FOUNDATION OF EFFECTIVE HEALTHCARE TEAMS

When patients place their trust in us, they're not just relying on our clinical skills — they're depending on the strength of the entire team behind those skills. Trust is what allows healthcare teams to function as a unified whole, especially in high-stakes, emotionally charged environments. It's what enables us to navigate complexity with confidence, compassion, and clarity.

But trust isn't built on qualifications alone — it's built through emotional intelligence. The ability to understand and regulate our own emotions, while staying attuned to those of our teammates, creates the kind of psychological safety that allows people to show up fully, contribute honestly, and support each other through both routine and unpredictable moments. It's the everyday actions — showing up, listening well, following through, and acknowledging others — that quietly build trust over time. These interactions send a powerful message: "You matter. Your voice counts. We're in this together."

VULNERABILITY AND TRUST: NAVIGATING THE DELICATE BALANCE

Trust is built through vulnerability — the courage to admit when we're struggling, to ask for help, or to acknowledge a mistake without fear of judgement. But let's be honest: vulnerability can feel uncomfortable, especially in healthcare, where we're often expected to appear competent and composed at all times.

This is where emotional intelligence becomes essential. Teams that value empathy and connection over hierarchy and ego create space for people to be human. For example, I remember a story a physician friend shared with me. She was leading a team debrief after a particularly challenging shift in the ICU. One of the nurses, visibly shaken, admitted she had missed a critical observation earlier in the day. The room went quiet — but instead of shaming or blaming, the team thanked her for her honesty, talked through what had happened, and worked together to adjust their handover processes. That nurse walked away not defeated, but supported — and the whole team walked away stronger.

I try to bring that same energy into my own practice. Whether it's someone needing to reschedule a shift because of a personal issue or a team member owning up to a clinical misstep, I want them to know they'll be met with understanding, not judgement. Vulnerability, when supported, is one of the most powerful trust builders we have.

CONSISTENCY AND RELIABILITY: THE PILLARS OF TRUST

Unpredictability is natural part of healthcare. For this reason, consistency becomes a quiet anchor; the steady presence that helps team members feel secure and supported, even when the day is anything but. When people know what to expect from one another — emotionally, professionally, and behaviourally — it creates a sense of rhythm and stability. This predictability in how we show up allows everyone to focus less on navigating interpersonal uncertainty and more on doing their best work.

Consistency is about more than just routines — it's about emotional presence. It's being someone your team knows they can count on to keep their cool under pressure, communicate clearly, and follow through on what you say you'll do. It's about making decisions that are fair and values-aligned, even when they're not the easiest or most convenient. That kind of predictability builds trust, because it reassures people that they won't be blindsided or left guessing about how they'll be treated or what's expected of them.

Reliability complements consistency — it's the daily follow-through, the quiet showing up, and the delivery of what's needed, when it's needed. Yes, this includes technical competence and task completion, but it also encompasses emotional dependability. Are you the kind of colleague who notices when someone's had a tough morning and checks in? Do you remember what matters to your team — like how one of your dental assistants gets nervous on busy days and just needs a little reassurance at morning huddle?

These small, human gestures carry weight. In fact, they often speak louder than the big moments. When we remember a teammate's birthday, ask about their parent in hospital, or simply offer to take something off their plate without being asked — it sends the message: I see you, I care about you, and I've got your back.

This sense of reliability is reciprocal. Just as I aim to be a steady and supportive presence for my team, I also rely on them to bring the same level of care and commitment to their roles. Our receptionist sets the tone the moment a patient walks through the door. Our assistants know how I work and are already reaching for the next instrument before I ask. That shared rhythm, built over time through consistency and trust, transforms the flow of the day — it reduces friction, enhances communication, and allows us to operate as a cohesive unit, even under pressure.

Consistency and reliability don't mean we have to be perfect. We're all human — there will be off days, miscommunications, and mistakes. But what matters is how we respond. If I drop the ball, I own it. If someone on the team is struggling, we rally around them. This kind of dependable, values-driven culture is what makes trust stick. It's not just about meeting deadlines or performing well during a procedure — it's about showing up, every day, in ways that reinforce that we're all in this together.

TRUST AND PATIENT CARE: THE ULTIMATE GOAL

What happens inside the team is felt by those outside it. Patients are incredibly perceptive. They can tell when a team is in sync — and they can just as quickly sense when something's off. When patients witness open communication, mutual respect, and genuine support among their care team, they feel more confident, more relaxed, and more involved in their own care.

In teams built on trust, there's no hesitation to clarify instructions, ask questions, or admit when something's unclear. This transparency not only prevents mistakes — it enhances care quality, because everyone feels safe to speak up and collaborate.

I've also found that trust gives teams the resilience to bounce back from setbacks. When things don't go as planned, a high-trust team will come together to reflect, learn, and adjust — rather than pointing fingers or sweeping issues under the rug. That shared accountability is powerful. It's what helps us turn challenges into lessons, and lessons into stronger systems and relationships.

Trust isn't something that just happens — it's earned. It's built through daily interactions, emotional intelligence, and a shared commitment to doing our best for one another and our patients. In my experience, the most effective teams are not necessarily the ones with the fanciest tools or the most accolades — but the ones that know how to trust, communicate, and care for each other deeply. When we build that kind of team, everyone benefits — especially the people we're here to serve.

5.6 Navigating Conflict with Emotional Intelligence

> *"The behaviour of others may be a stimulus for our feelings, but not the cause. We are never angry because of what someone else did...It's not what the other person does, but the images and interpretations in my own head that produce my anger."*
>
> — Marshall Rosenberg

UTILISING SELF-AWARENESS AND EMPATHY TO DISCERN CONFLICT ROOTS

Every conflict is like an iceberg — what you see on the surface is often just a fraction of what lies beneath. Beneath every disagreement are complex emotions, unmet needs, and differing perspectives. Navigating these layers requires two critical components of emotional intelligence: self-awareness and empathy.

Self-awareness is about being able to observe your own thoughts, emotions, and behaviours without judgment. It's recognising your emotional triggers and biases, and understanding how these influence the way you respond in challenging situations. For instance, if you find yourself feeling defensive during a disagreement, instead of immediately reacting, it helps to pause and ask yourself: "What's really going on here?" Is this reaction coming from the current situation, or is it tapping into a past experience or a deeper insecurity? Maybe you've had a similar disagreement before that left you feeling dismissed, or perhaps being questioned makes you feel like your competence is under threat. Identifying those emotional undercurrents in real time isn't always easy, but it's powerful. That pause — that brief moment of reflection — gives you the chance to respond thoughtfully rather than react impulsively. Over time, these small moments of self-reflection help you develop emotional agility, allowing you to stay grounded and intentional even when emotions are running high. And when you're able to do that, you create space not just for better outcomes, but for deeper connection and mutual respect in your relationships — whether with patients, team members, or yourself.

Pairing this introspection with empathy is where real growth happens. Once you've taken a moment to check in with your own emotional response, the next step is to shift your focus outward and step into the other person's shoes. Empathy allows you to move beyond assumptions and really consider what might be driving their behaviour. Maybe a team member seems defensive or resistant to feedback — but instead of interpreting that as disrespect or unwillingness to improve, empathy encourages you to pause and ask, "What might be going on for them right now?" They might be feeling overwhelmed, insecure, or like their efforts haven't been recognised. When you approach the situation with curiosity rather than judgment, you're far more likely to open a meaningful dialogue — one that builds trust instead of tearing it down.

This dual approach — introspection paired with empathy — transforms conflict from something adversarial into something collaborative. It shifts the dynamic from "Who's right?" to "What's really going on here, and how can we move forward together?" It helps you address the root cause rather than just the surface issue, which is critical if you want to avoid resentment building up and festering beneath the surface. When both parties feel seen, heard, and understood, resolution becomes less about compromise and more about genuine understanding.

SAFEGUARDING PROFESSIONAL RELATIONSHIPS AMIDST DISAGREEMENTS

Conflict can easily put strain on professional relationships. Preserving those vital connections during moments of disagreement requires a blend of assertiveness and compassion — but it also presents a key leadership opportunity. When you approach conflict with emotional intelligence, you're not just resolving an issue — you're modelling the kind of behaviour that shapes team norms. Over time, your team learns that it's possible to have hard conversations with respect, clarity, and care. This is where emotional intelligence becomes so important — it allows you to express your views clearly and firmly while still showing respect and empathy for the other person's perspective.

A simple but powerful tool here is the use of "I" statements. As a leader, when you open with "I feel concerned when deadlines aren't met because it impacts patient care," you're modelling emotional ownership — and you're setting a cultural precedent that owning our impact is how we solve problems together. It also helps communicate your feelings and the implications of the situation without casting blame or triggering defensiveness. This approach stands in stark contrast to "you" statements, which often sound accusatory and can escalate tensions. For instance, saying, "You never meet deadlines, and it's causing problems," shifts the focus onto the other person's perceived shortcomings, potentially putting them on the defensive and closing off productive dialogue. "I" statements help keep the focus on the impact of the issue rather than turning it into a personal attack. They create just enough distance to keep the conversation constructive, while still being honest and direct. This method not only keeps the focus on the issue at hand but also fosters an atmosphere of respect and mutual understanding, setting the tone for a collaborative resolution.

As we've touched on a few times now, active listening is another crucial strategy. When you make a genuine effort to hear not just someone's words but the emotion behind them, it shows that you value their experience. If a colleague is upset about a sudden change in the schedule, for example, simply saying "I can see this is frustrating for you" goes a long way. It shows empathy, creates space for conversation, and defuses tension before it escalates.

As leaders, our communication style ultimately sets the tone. When we use tools like "I" statements or reflective listening in tense moments, we're coaching our teams — subtly but powerfully — on how to navigate disagreement constructively. This helps embed a culture where conflict doesn't mean rupture, but rather, an opportunity for growth and collaboration. Preserving relationships during conflict doesn't mean avoiding disagreement — it means handling it with emotional maturity. And often, when these conversations are approached with openness and respect, the relationship actually grows stronger as a result. It signals to the other person that you're committed to working through challenges together, not walking away from them. That kind of trust is what solid, resilient teams are built on.

Reflection: How Do You Show Up During Conflict?

Think back to a difficult conversation you've had in the past — or take a moment after your next challenging conversation or disagreement — to reflect on the following:

- *Did I express myself clearly without blaming or shaming?*
- *Did I use "I" statements to describe how I felt and why?*

- *Did I pause to really listen — not just to the words, but to the emotion behind them?*
- *Did I stay open and curious about the other person's perspective?*
- *Was my tone respectful and calm, even when I felt frustrated?*
- *What could I do differently next time to strengthen the relationship, not just resolve the issue?*

Remember: conflict handled with care can actually build trust, not break it. Every conversation is an opportunity to model the kind of culture we want in our teams — one that values empathy, clarity, and mutual respect.

EMBRACING CONFLICT AS A CATALYST FOR TEAM DYNAMICS ENHANCEMENT

Conflict often gets a bad rap — but it doesn't have to be a negative force. When handled with emotional intelligence, disagreements can become powerful springboards for growth, innovation, and stronger team dynamics. It all starts with reframing conflict — not as a battle to win, but as a shared problem to solve.

Take a situation where two team members have different ideas about how to streamline patient intake. Tension starts to rise, and left unchecked, it could easily snowball into resentment or silence. But instead of avoiding the issue or letting it simmer, a leader who practices emotional intelligence can step in — not to take sides, but to facilitate a respectful, open conversation. By guiding the discussion toward the shared goal — improving the patient experience — both perspectives can be explored without judgment. Often, what starts as conflict ends in a better process and a stronger sense of ownership and teamwork.

I've seen this happen many times in my own clinic. When we lean into conflict instead of sweeping it under the rug, it often leads to creative solutions we wouldn't have come up with on our own. More often than not, each person comes into a disagreement with their own fixed idea of how a problem should be solved. But when we take the time to truly listen, understand each other's perspectives, and work through the issue together, we often discover a third option — a win-win solution that neither side had considered on their own. It's this process of collaboration that not only resolves the issue but also strengthens the team. And more than that, it deepens our understanding of each other. When people feel truly heard — even in disagreement — it builds trust. And that trust becomes the glue that holds a team together, especially when things get hard.

DE-ESCALATING TENSE SITUATIONS: SIMPLE SHIFTS WITH BIG IMPACT

Sometimes, despite our best efforts, conflict finds us. Emotions run high, misunderstandings escalate, and before you know it, you're in a tense situation that feels like it could go sideways fast. That's when de-escalation becomes essential — not just for resolving the issue at hand, but for preserving trust and keeping relationships intact.

One of the most underrated but powerful tools in these moments is the deliberate pause. I'm not talking about storming off or going silent out of frustration. I mean a purposeful, emotionally intelligent pause — a brief moment to collect your thoughts and allow everyone's nervous systems a chance to regulate. It might be just a few seconds of silence, taking a deep breath or saying something like, "Can we take a moment to regroup before we continue?" But that small interruption in the heat of the moment can completely change the trajectory of the conversation.

When emotions are heightened, logic tends to go out the window. People stop listening and start defending. A pause interrupts that spiral and gives space for more considered, compassionate communication. I've seen it work time and time again, both in clinical settings and team meetings — whether it's a tough conversation about performance or a disagreement about patient care. That reset moment gives everyone a chance to breathe and come back to the table in a more grounded way.

Even more effective? Pair the pause with a simple calming technique. Step outside for a breath of fresh air, do a few rounds of box breathing, or just take a slow walk to the breakroom and back. These are small, practical things we can all do to reset in a high-stress moment. And when we model this behaviour as leaders, it normalises emotional regulation for everyone around us.

Another powerful technique is to acknowledge the other person's emotions. You don't have to agree with their point of view but recognising how they feel can be incredibly disarming. A statement like, "I can see this is really frustrating for you," or "It sounds like this has been weighing on you," signals that you're listening and trying to understand. That little moment of validation can bring the temperature down significantly.

That said, it's worth being mindful of how these acknowledgments can sometimes come across. Saying "I understand" can sometimes feel dismissive if it's not genuine or if the other person feels misunderstood. Instead, phrases like "I can imagine that was tough", "I appreciate how difficult this must feel" or "I respect the effort you've put into this" tend to land better. They offer empathy without overstepping or pretending to know exactly what the other person is going through.

Language really does matter in these situations. Even a tiny word like "but" can derail the whole tone of a conversation and you risk the loss of connection.

Consider the difference between:

- "I really appreciate all the work you've done *but* we need to change direction,"

vs.

- "I really appreciate all the work you've done, *and* I want to explore how we can move forward in a way that works for both of us."

That one-word shift keeps the acknowledgment intact and invites collaboration instead of contradiction. We need to be careful not to inadvertently negate the acknowledgement and undermine our efforts to build or maintain rapport.

Another technique I love is reframing the conflict — shifting the focus from blame to shared problem-solving. Instead of saying, "You're not pulling your weight," you might say, "We're finding it tough to stay on top of the workload — what do you think might help?" It's subtle, but it changes the entire energy of the conversation. It becomes less about who's at fault and more about how we can work together to improve things.

I had a recent example in my own clinic. One of my team members had been consistently falling behind on admin tasks. Instead of sitting them down and listing out everything they hadn't done (which likely would've put them on the defensive), I opened with, "I've noticed things seem a little overwhelming at the moment — what's going on, and how can I support you?" That small shift created space for a much more honest conversation. We uncovered a couple of workflow bottlenecks that were easily fixed and avoided what could've become an ongoing point of frustration.

The bottom line? De-escalation is not about backing down. It's about staying connected — even when emotions are high — so that we can move forward with mutual respect and understanding. A few intentional shifts in language, body language, and tone can make all the difference in keeping conversations productive and relationships intact. Whether it's a heated moment or a quiet simmer of frustration, how we show up in conflict sets the tone for the entire team. By bringing emotional intelligence into these moments, we don't just prevent breakdowns — we build stronger, more resilient relationships.

GO-TO PHRASES FOR DIFFICULT CONVERSATIONS

To make these strategies easier to apply in the moment, I've created a simple visual reference with some of the phrases I come back to time and time again. These aren't scripts — but they can act as gentle cues to help you approach tough conversations with clarity and care.

Go-to Phrases for Difficult Conversations

Reframe Statements

Shifts the focus towards collaboration

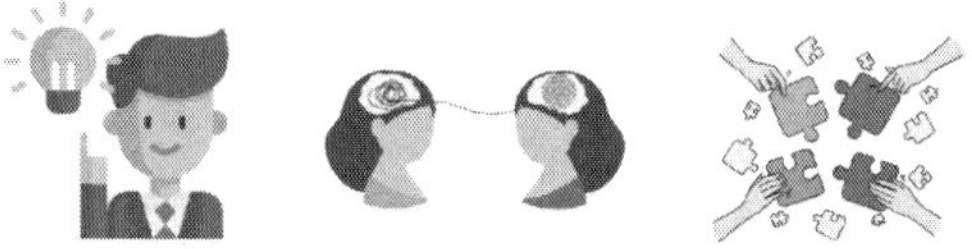

"I'd like to understand more about..." | "What do you think we can do about this?" | "How can we work through this together?"

I - Statements

Communicates personal experience and concern

"I noticed that..." | "I'm feeling..." | "I'd appreciate your help with..."

Empathy Openers

Acknowledges the other person's feelings

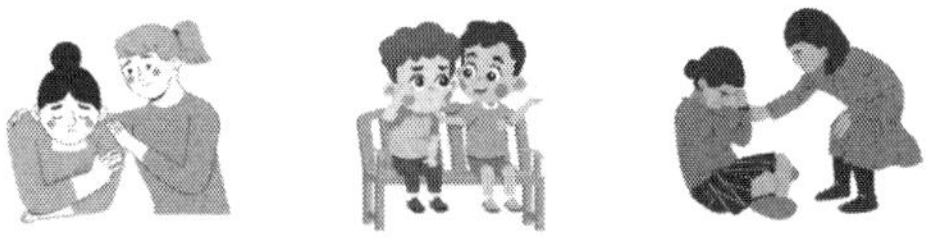

"I can see that this is hard for you..." | "It sounds like you're feeling..." | "I can imagine that was difficult..."

Always remember to: Pause and Acknowledge

Creates space to defuse tension

Keep this list somewhere accessible — on your desk, in your notes app, or shared with your team. Sometimes, just having the right words ready can make all the difference in staying calm, connected, and constructive during high-stakes conversations.

While many conflicts can be resolved with emotional intelligence and strong communication, some tensions run deeper — especially when they stem from ongoing challenges with a colleague. In these cases, our ability to stay emotionally grounded and lead with clarity becomes even more essential. Let's explore what it looks like to navigate these dynamics thoughtfully and protect both team culture and professional wellbeing.

5.7 Dealing with Difficult Colleagues Through Understanding

"In the middle of difficulty lies opportunity."

— Albert Einstein

Healthcare teams are built from diverse personalities, experiences, and communication styles — which is a strength, but also means we'll occasionally encounter colleagues who challenge us. Add the pressure of high-stakes patient care, and minor tensions can sometimes escalate into professional obstacles. While these situations can be frustrating, they are also opportunities for growth — both personally and as a team.

The first step in addressing challenges in order to improve a strained relationship with a colleague is empathy. Empathy doesn't mean excusing bad behaviour but rather seeking to understand what might be driving it. Instead of focusing on how their behaviour is impacting you, consider what they might be experiencing. Instead of labelling their actions as purely "difficult," take a moment to ask yourself: What might be causing this? Are they stressed? Feeling unsupported? Struggling with personal or professional challenges? Approaching the situation with genuine curiosity — without judgment — can shift your perspective.

This mindset allows you to reframe difficult behaviour — not as a personal attack, but as a response to unmet needs or unresolved frustration. For example, a colleague who snaps at others during meetings might be struggling with workloads that feel overwhelming. By engaging with them empathetically — without judgment — you open the door to a deeper understanding and potentially resolving the tension. A simple conversation like, "You seemed really frustrated earlier — are you okay? Is there anything I can do to help?" can go a long way in diffusing conflict and showing them that you care.

CLEAR AND CONSTRUCTIVE COMMUNICATION

Open, honest communication is critical when dealing with workplace tensions. Emotional intelligence helps ensure that these conversations are direct yet respectful, striking a balance that allows both parties to feel heard.

Active listening is a key part of this. It's about truly focusing on the other person — what they're saying, how they're saying it, and the emotions behind their words — without rushing to formulate a response. For example, if a colleague is critical of your work, instead of reacting defensively, listen fully. You might say, "I hear that you're frustrated — can you help me understand what's concerning you so we can work through it?" This kind of response opens the door to problem-solving rather than escalating conflict.

Clear communication also means being assertive about your needs. Use "I" statements to express how their behaviour affects you without assigning blame. For example: "I feel overwhelmed when tasks are reassigned at the last minute without discussion — it makes it harder for me to manage my priorities. Could we agree on a process to handle this going forward?". Instead of saying, "You're always interrupting me during meetings," try, "I feel unheard when I'm interrupted, and I'd really appreciate it if we could find a way to ensure everyone gets their turn to contribute." This approach keeps the focus on resolving the issue rather than escalating it. These conversations may feel uncomfortable at first, but they lay the groundwork for a healthier, more collaborative relationship.

ESTABLISHING AND MAINTAINING BOUNDARIES

Boundaries are vital for preserving your well-being and creating a productive work environment. In the context of difficult colleagues, boundaries help define acceptable behaviour and clarify expectations for how you interact professionally.

Setting boundaries starts with self-awareness — understanding what you're willing to tolerate and where you draw the line. For example, if a colleague habitually interrupts your focus with unnecessary demands, it's okay to say, "I'd like to help, but I need to finish this task first. Can we schedule a time to discuss this later?" It's not about being uncooperative but about protecting your time and energy so you can work effectively. If a colleague repeatedly sends work tasks after hours, it's okay to communicate your limits: "I value being responsive, but I also need to maintain my personal time. Can we discuss a system for managing non-urgent requests outside of work hours?" While we noted earlier how "and" can preserve connection, in these cases, using "but" helps reinforce the boundary in a respectful, clear way — signalling that while you're willing to help, there's a limit that needs to be acknowledged.

Once boundaries are set, they need to be upheld consistently. This might feel uncomfortable at first, especially in collaborative, service-oriented environments where helping others is the norm. But holding your boundaries — kindly and clearly — sends a strong message of mutual respect. It shows your colleagues that while you value teamwork, you also prioritise healthy, balanced interactions. Over time, consistency builds trust; people come to understand where the lines are and are more likely to respect them. And when you model this behaviour, you also give others permission to do the same — contributing to a healthier, more sustainable work culture overall.

MEDIATION FOR CONFLICT RESOLUTION

Sometimes, despite your best efforts, conflicts remain unresolved. In these cases, seeking mediation can be a constructive next step. Mediation isn't about "winning" an argument; it's about finding common ground with the help of a neutral third party. In larger organisations, this might involve a supervisor or HR professional. In smaller clinics without formal HR departments, it could be a trusted senior team member, practice manager, or even an external mediator brought in to help facilitate the conversation. What matters most is creating a psychologically safe space where both parties can share their perspectives and work toward a constructive solution.

For example, a mediator might help structure a conversation where each person outlines their concerns, and together you agree on strategies to improve communication or address ongoing issues. Mediation reinforces the idea that resolving conflict isn't about assigning blame but about preserving the professional relationships that underpin quality patient care.

WHEN DIFFICULT BEHAVIOUR BECOMES DISRUPTIVE

Despite your best efforts to address issues with a difficult colleague, there may come a time when their behaviour continues to disrupt the team. It's important to recognise that one person's bad attitude or persistent negativity can significantly affect the morale of the entire group. A single toxic presence can create friction between team members, leading to a tense atmosphere that patients will inevitably sense, potentially affecting their experience and trust in the care provided.

In these situations, as much as we want to resolve conflicts and preserve relationships, it's critical to prioritise the well-being of the team and the organisation. Not every person is the right fit for every workplace culture, and this applies to both new hires and long-standing team members — especially as the company evolves and grows.

When it becomes clear that someone's behaviour is consistently misaligned with the values and culture of the organisation, it may be necessary to make a difficult decision for the greater good. This could mean transitioning them to a role within the organisation that better suits their strengths or, in some cases, letting them go altogether. While this step can feel uncomfortable, it's often the best outcome not only for the team but for the individual as well. They may thrive in a different environment that better aligns with their personality and professional goals.

As leaders — formal or informal — our responsibility isn't to please everyone at the expense of the team, but to foster a culture where empathy, accountability, and alignment coexist. Sometimes, the greatest act of leadership is making the hard call with both compassion and clarity. Protecting the team culture isn't just important — it's essential. A positive, cohesive team is far better equipped to deliver exceptional care, collaborate effectively, and create an environment where everyone — including patients — feels supported and valued. In some cases, the most compassionate choice for all involved is to part ways and allow everyone to move forward in a more constructive direction.

5.8 Servant Leadership: Leading with Heart, Not Ego

"Leadership is not about being in charge. Leadership is about taking care of those in your charge."

— Simon Sinek

Building on the emotional intelligence skills we've already explored, servant leadership brings these qualities to life in how we lead, serve, and support our teams. Leadership is far more than a title — it's a responsibility to inspire, empower, and cultivate a positive workplace culture. At the heart of that influence lies emotional intelligence and a deep sense of service — two essential tools for navigating the complexities of high-stakes environments like healthcare. To lead effectively, we can't just manage tasks or people; we need to genuinely connect with our teams, build resilience, and guide with intention and purpose.

This philosophy is beautifully captured in the concept of servant leadership — a model that prioritises empowering others, fostering meaningful relationships, and creating a culture where collaboration, compassion, and growth thrive. It's the leadership style I strive to embody in both my life and my clinical practice.

LEADING BY SERVING

Servant leadership is all about flipping the traditional leadership model on its head. Rather than focusing on authority, control, or climbing to the top, it's about leading with the mindset of service — putting the needs of your team, your patients, and those around you first. Originally introduced by Robert K. Greenleaf, this philosophy challenges the old-school hierarchy where power flows from the top down. Instead, servant leadership is about support flowing from the bottom up — leaders lifting others so they can reach their full potential.

For me, this leadership style just makes sense. It's not about being the boss or having all the answers — it's about creating an environment where people feel safe, empowered, and supported to do their best work. The core values behind it — authenticity, honest communication, integrity, compassion, empowerment, continuous learning, and putting others before self — are the same values that build trust and connection in any strong relationship. And when these values are embedded in the way we lead, they create workplaces where collaboration thrives, morale lifts, and innovation is possible.

TRADITIONAL LEADERSHIP VS. SERVANT LEADERSHIP

In more traditional models of leadership, success is often tied to control and authority. Leaders are expected to direct from the top, drive results, and stay focused on output. Often, it's a style that leaves little room for collaboration — and can unintentionally create an environment where team members feel unheard or undervalued. The leader ends up doing most of the talking, and people can start to feel like they're just there to follow orders.

Servant leadership stands in stark contrast to that approach. It's not about power — it's about service. Servant leaders understand that their role is to support and elevate others. They measure success not by what they accomplish personally, but by how well their team grows, develops, and thrives. They listen more than they speak, ask more than they instruct, and lead with humility rather than ego.

Personally, I've always believed that no leader should ever be "too good" to get involved at any level. Whether it's jumping in to help at the front desk during a busy period, checking in on how someone's really doing, or simply pitching in wherever needed — those moments matter. They show your team that you're in it with them, not above them. The most effective leaders I've seen (and the kind I try to be) are the ones who create an atmosphere of shared purpose, remove obstacles where they can, and make sure everyone feels seen, supported, and part of something bigger.

THE CHARACTERISTIC OF SERVANT LEADERS

Servant leadership is built on a set of defining characteristics, each aligning with building trust, fostering collaboration, and prioritising the well-being of others. True servant leadership begins and ends with the heart — with a focus on humility, empathy, and lifting others up. These six core values form the HEARTS of a great servant leader:

H – Humility

A servant leader leads with modesty, knowing that success is a team effort. They never act like they're above others and are always willing to step in wherever needed. They prioritise the contributions of others and give credit where it's due.

E – Empowerment

They support their team to grow, develop, and shine — mentoring and guiding them to reach their full potential while also celebrating their wins along the way.

A – Authenticity

They show up as their true selves, building trust through honesty and consistency — in how they speak, act, and relate to others, whether professionally, publicly, or personally.

R – Responsibility

Servant leaders take ownership — not just of outcomes, but of creating an environment where people feel safe, supported, and valued. They hold themselves and others accountable with fairness and care.

T – Trust & Tolerance

They foster psychological safety and mutual respect, listening openly and accepting others' perspectives, even when they differ from their own.

S – Stewardship

They lead with purpose above personal gain, acting in service of the greater good — of the team, the patients, and the organisation. This includes taking risks, innovating, and confronting challenges with integrity and courage.

For me, one of the simplest yet most impactful habits is regularly checking in with my team: "How are you going? Is there anything I can do to help you?" It's a small gesture, but it reminds people that I'm here to support them, not just manage them. That's what leading with HEARTS looks like.

PRACTICING SERVANT LEADERSHIP

Being a servant leader doesn't mean lowering your standards — it means pairing high expectations with compassion, support, and clear communication. I love the quote by Neil Strauss: "*Unspoken expectations are premeditated resentments.*" That line hits hard because it's so true. If we expect excellence from our team — which we should, especially if it's one of our core values — we need to be just as clear about what excellence looks like. It's our job to articulate expectations and provide the guidance and tools people need to meet them. That's not being soft; it's being fair.

Servant leadership is really about how we show up for our people. And just to be clear — it's not about being a pushover or avoiding tough conversations or decisions. It's not about hierarchy or holding onto power. It's about service, support, and stewardship. It's about balancing accountability with empathy, holding the team — and yourself — to a high standard while creating an environment where people feel safe, supported, and encouraged to grow.

There are tangible ways to bring this to life every day. The acronym LEADS captures five key ways to put servant leadership into action:

L – Learn Who Your Team Really Is

Get to know your team members beyond their job descriptions. What are their goals, both personal and professional? What motivates and energises them? What stresses them out? When you take the time to understand them as individuals — not just workers — you can lead more effectively. Tools like personality testing (e.g. DISC, Myers-Briggs, or Clifton Strengths) can be incredibly useful here. They help you understand communication preferences, working styles, and even stress triggers, which ultimately allows you to support and communicate with your team more thoughtfully.

E – Eliminate Barriers

Sometimes people underperform not because they don't care, but because they're navigating hidden obstacles. It might be a clunky process, a lack of clarity, or even an unresolved interpersonal issue. It's our responsibility as leaders to identify and remove these roadblocks. Regular one-on-one check-ins are a great opportunity to ask, "What's getting in your way right now, and how can I help clear the path?"

A – Acknowledge and Appreciate

Never underestimate the power of a genuine thank you. Recognition doesn't have to be grand or formal. Often, a quick moment of appreciation — a few kind words in a team meeting or a thoughtful message — can make someone feel seen and valued. And beyond praise, remember to acknowledge life's big (and small) moments for your team. Whether it's a birthday, work anniversary, family challenge or personal win, showing that you care strengthens connection, boosts morale, and builds long-term loyalty.

D – Discover What Matters

Great leaders listen for what *really* matters to their people. Ask questions like, "What does success look like for you?" or "What's one thing I can do to support you this month?" These small conversations build a culture of openness. It also means you're less likely to be blindsided by someone quietly struggling or disengaging.

S – Support Growth and Accountability

Servant leadership is not about being everyone's best friend or avoiding tough conversations. On the contrary — it's about balancing support with accountability. Hold yourself and your team to a high standard, but do it in a way that's kind, constructive, and future-focused. If someone drops the ball, address it directly, but also explore what support they might need to do better next time. People don't grow in fear-based environments — they grow when they feel safe, seen, and supported.

At the heart of all of this is emotional intelligence. It's what helps you read the room, respond with empathy, and tailor your leadership to the needs of the people around you. These leaders listen more than they speak, approach problems with a calm and open mind, and recognise the power of vulnerability and authenticity in building trust. When your team knows you care about them — not just their output — they'll go above and beyond because they feel connected to the work and the bigger mission behind it.

THE RIPPLE EFFECT

Servant leadership has a profound, cascading impact. As Roy T. Bennett famously said, "*Great leaders create more leaders, not followers.*" When you lead by serving, you don't just influence the task at hand — you empower others to step up, take ownership, and lead in their own way. That's how culture is built — not through control, but through example.

This ripple effect transforms teams into cohesive, collaborative units that value empathy, accountability, and a shared purpose. But for this to really take hold, every team member needs to be crystal clear on the mission and vision of the organisation. People can't align with what they don't understand. When your team knows not just *what* you do but *why* you do it, they're more likely to feel invested, make aligned decisions, and take meaningful ownership of their role within the bigger picture.

Emotionally intelligent leadership amplifies this effect. When a leader leads with emotional intelligence — by listening, validating, and responding with empathy — they create an environment where people feel safe, valued, and heard. In a healthcare setting, this emotional safety becomes the foundation for collaboration and trust. Team members are more likely to speak up about concerns, offer ideas, and support one another — especially when things get stressful. This kind of open communication isn't just nice to have — it directly prevents errors and improves patient outcomes.

In high-pressure situations, emotionally intelligent teams are better equipped to stay calm and focused. Instead of getting swept up in the stress, they lean into their training and the trust they've built with each other. They know they can rely on one another. They're not just reacting — they're responding with intention and care. That has a powerful impact on patient trust and safety. Relationship-centred care becomes not just an ideal, but something that consistently plays out in real life.

There's also a deeper shift that happens when leaders consistently model EQ. Over time, the team starts to reflect those behaviours back — not just to the leader, but to one another. They become more self-aware, more empathetic, and more capable of handling conflict or setbacks constructively. That's the real magic of this style of leadership: it multiplies. One person's emotional intelligence can spark growth across an entire team.

As these values take root, the collective emotional intelligence of the organisation strengthens. Burnout decreases. Job satisfaction improves. People feel like they belong — and when people feel like they belong, they show up more fully and consistently for their patients and for each other.

5.9 Motivation and Recognition: The Emotional Fuel for Thriving Teams

---

> *"The deepest principle in human nature is the craving to be appreciated."*
>
> — William James

EMPATHY AS A LEADERSHIP TOOL

Empathy is hands down one of the most powerful tools a leader can have — and yet, it's so often overlooked in favour of strategy, efficiency, or control. But the truth is, without empathy, all the other pieces fall flat. Empathy allows us to lead with a human lens — to step outside of our own perspective and really understand what someone else is experiencing.

In leadership, this isn't just about being "nice." It's about tuning in. Empathetic leaders notice when something's off, pick up on emotional cues, and ask the right questions. They don't shy away from discomfort or hard conversations — instead, they lean in with compassion, curiosity, and a willingness to help. That kind of presence creates the deep trust and respect that strong, motivated teams are built on.

Take, for example, a team member who's usually upbeat and efficient but suddenly seems distracted, short-tempered, or withdrawn. An empathetic leader doesn't ignore it or write it off as laziness or disinterest. Instead, they create a safe moment to check in: "Hey, I've noticed you haven't seemed like yourself lately. Is everything okay? Do you want to talk about it?" Sometimes that conversation opens the door to a personal struggle the team member has been carrying quietly. Other times, it might be work-related stress or even miscommunication with a colleague. Either way, showing genuine interest in what's going on beneath the surface makes people feel seen — and that in itself is incredibly motivating.

When empathy is part of your leadership style, your team doesn't just feel managed — they feel genuinely cared for. And people who feel cared for show up differently. They're more engaged, more loyal, and more likely to go the extra mile not out of obligation, but out of connection and purpose. This sense of loyalty is one of the most powerful — and often underestimated — benefits of emotionally intelligent leadership. When people feel safe, seen, and supported, they're far more likely to stay. In a field like healthcare, where turnover can disrupt continuity of care, increase recruitment costs, and place strain on the rest of the team, long-term retention isn't just a nice-to-have — it's essential. A stable team creates a sense of rhythm and familiarity that helps everything run more smoothly, from internal communication to patient experience. Loyalty also strengthens culture: over time, people who stay grow together, learn from one another, and build a collective memory that becomes the bedrock of trust, collaboration, and shared purpose.

Empathy also invites collaboration. When team members feel like their perspectives matter, they're more likely to contribute ideas, voice concerns, and take initiative. It transforms your clinic from a place people show up to work into a space where they feel they belong. A great example of this was the day a dental company rep visited us to demonstrate the CEREC machine — a piece of technology that allows us to design and create crowns in-house. At the time, I hadn't been considering it for the practice — it was a significant investment, and not something that was on my radar. But my dental assistant and practice manager saw the potential immediately. They were excited, curious, and asked if they could arrange an in-clinic demo. Their initiative and passion for what this could mean for our patients and workflow really struck me. Their enthusiasm was contagious, and ultimately, it was their belief in the idea that convinced me to move forward. It's since become one of the best investments we've ever made. That kind of innovation and progress wouldn't have happened without a team that felt safe, empowered, and genuinely invested in the future of the practice.

Of course, empathy isn't about fixing everyone's problems or taking on the emotional load of the entire team. It's about leading with heart, listening without judgment, and holding space for others while still guiding the team forward. It's that balance of kindness and clarity, of support and standards, that defines true emotionally intelligent leadership. In my own practice, I've found that the moments where I've led with empathy — especially when someone is struggling — have been some of the most powerful. They don't just build trust; they inspire people to rise. And that, to me, is what leadership is all about: lifting others up so they can do their best work, feel proud of their contribution, and go home at the end of the day knowing they matter.

CRAFTING A VISION WITH EMOTIONAL CONNECTION

A great leader doesn't just manage tasks — they inspire their team by painting a compelling vision of the future. When that vision resonates emotionally, it aligns with the team's values and aspirations, creating a shared sense of purpose that goes beyond day-to-day responsibilities.

At Corner 32 Dental, our philosophy, mission, and vision serve as the foundation for this emotional connection. We're not just in the business of dentistry — we're in the business of transforming lives and changing perceptions about dental care. By providing exceptional and compassionate dental care through focusing on the mouth-body connection and creating a truly unique patient experience, we ensure that overall well-being is at the heart of everything we do. Over the past decade, we've combined state-of-the-art technology with personalised care to enhance thousands of smiles, improve the health and happiness of our community, and become multi-award-winning industry leaders.

When I share this philosophy with my team, I'm not just reciting statements — I'm inviting them to be part of a movement. For instance, our mission to provide exceptional dental care that transforms the way people feel about visiting the dentist by delivering relationship-centred, high-quality treatment and a truly unique patient experience to 10,000 patients by 2030 isn't just a number. It's a reminder of the real lives we touch every day. It's about every adult who overcomes their fear of the dentist, every child who begins their dental journey on a positive note to prevent dental anxiety later in life, and every individual whose quality of life improves because we helped them prioritise their health.

Our vision — to create a dental practice renowned for redefining dental care by creating a compassionate, patient-first experience that transforms smiles and changes lives, making the world a healthier and happier place — is proudly displayed in our office and serves as a constant reminder of our purpose. It's a vision that goes beyond the technical aspects of dentistry, inspiring each team member to see their role as pivotal in creating a healthier, happier world.

One way this vision comes to life is through storytelling. Sharing real-life examples of how we've helped patients achieve not only better dental health but also a renewed sense of self-confidence reminds the team of the "why" behind their work. Whether it's a patient who overcame years of dental anxiety or someone who can now smile freely after years of discomfort, these stories resonate deeply. By connecting our daily efforts to these bigger goals, we energise our team to push through challenges and continuously strive for excellence. This vision isn't just a directive — it's a rallying cry. It reminds us that our work matters and that together, we're making a tangible difference in the lives of our patients and our community.

When leaders take the time to craft and communicate a clear vision, they do more than just set direction — they create a shared sense of purpose that inspires and unites the entire team. Suddenly, everyone — from the front desk to the treatment room — can see how their individual role contributes to something bigger. That emotional connection to a common goal is what transforms a good team into an exceptional one.

If you haven't already defined your organisation's mission and vision — or if you haven't clearly communicated it to your team — now is the time. Because when people understand the "why" behind their work, they become motivated and energised to do their best.

RECOGNISING AND APPRECIATING CONTRIBUTIONS

Recognition and appreciation aren't just about good manners or ticking a leadership box — they're about letting people know they matter. It's easy to get caught up in what still needs to be done and forget to pause and celebrate what has already been achieved. But when someone feels genuinely seen and valued for their effort — not just for the outcome, but for the way they showed up — it fuels their sense of purpose and motivates them to keep going, especially during the tough days.

The most meaningful recognition is specific and personal. It's not just "Great job!" — it's "I really appreciated how patient and calm you were with that anxious patient this morning. You made a big difference to their experience." It's about noticing the *how*, not just the *what*.

For example, I'll often leave a handwritten note or send a message after a long day, just to acknowledge the resilience, kindness, or teamwork someone showed. A few heartfelt words like, "I saw how you stayed back to help the assistant clean up today — it didn't go unnoticed," can mean more than any grand gesture. Or, when the team hits a milestone — like getting through a busy week or receiving great feedback from a patient — I'll bring in morning tea, or we'll take a moment to celebrate it together.

Recently, I wasn't in the clinic because I was attending a course, and one of my associate dentists — a relatively new graduate — was treating a child with a badly decayed tooth. She tried everything she could to save it, but ultimately, it needed to be extracted. The child became distressed, and understandably, so did she. She wasn't able to get the tooth out, and the team ended up calling my other associate to see if she could come in and help. She did — without hesitation. Not only did she step in, but she also stayed afterwards to debrief with the new grad, offering tips, reassurance, and support. When I found out what had happened, I messaged her to say thank you. Her reply said everything: "Of course — we all know what that first year is like." That moment captured so much of what I value in a team: compassion, initiative, and a deep understanding that we're all in this together.

These small but consistent acts of appreciation build emotional safety and belonging. They remind people that they're not just a cog in the machine — they're a valued and essential part of a team that cares. And in my experience, when people feel appreciated, they become more engaged, more invested, and more willing to go the extra mile — not because they have to, but because they want to.

FOSTERING A CULTURE OF INSPIRATION AND MOTIVATION

Creating a workplace culture that genuinely inspires and motivates doesn't happen by accident — it's something that must be cultivated with care, intention, and consistency.

It starts with communication. In truly inspiring work cultures, open dialogue isn't just encouraged — it's expected. Ideas can be shared without fear of judgment, questions are welcomed, and feedback flows both ways. Leaders model this through their everyday interactions: they take the time to genuinely listen, respond calmly under pressure, and show a real interest in their team's growth and well-being. It's these subtle behaviours, repeated consistently, that shape the emotional tone of the team.

Motivated teams are often the result of leaders who empower rather than micromanage. They entrust team members with responsibilities that stretch them just enough — providing challenge, but not overwhelm — and then offer the support, guidance, and encouragement needed to succeed. A crucial part of this is setting people up for success, not failure. Delegating tasks without proper training, resources, or clarity can leave team members feeling lost, unsupported, and ultimately defeated. But when we take the time to prepare them properly — through mentoring, clear expectations, and check-ins along the way — we show that we're invested in their growth, not just the outcome.

When a team member expresses interest in learning a new skill or taking on a different responsibility, a strong leader will lean into that opportunity — whether it's supporting them through a course, pairing them with a mentor, or simply giving them the space and encouragement to step up with guidance in their back pocket. These moments don't just build capability — they build confidence, trust, and a sense of personal investment in the success of the team. And when people feel supported to rise to the occasion, they usually do.

A great example of this from my own practice is when my practice manager expressed an interest in designing and fabricating crowns herself using our new CEREC machine. She'd never done anything like that before, but I could see how enthusiastic she was about learning. I signed her up for courses, gave her the time and space to practice, and encouraged her every step of the way. That one opportunity added an entirely new dimension to her role. It gave her an outlet for her creativity, a renewed sense of purpose, and a whole lot of pride in being part of the clinical outcome. Now, every time she designs a beautiful crown, not only does the patient appreciate it — but she does too. She's built something with her own hands that contributes meaningfully to someone's health and confidence. And that kind of ownership? It's a game changer.

Equally important is how we respond when things don't go as planned. Great leaders don't see mistakes as failures — they see them as learning moments. They create space for the team to reflect together, asking questions like, "What worked?", "What didn't?", and "What can we do differently next time?" I've found that when a leader shows they're not afraid of things going wrong, it encourages the team to be brave and take thoughtful risks — because they know they won't be shamed for trying.

This kind of emotional safety is what drives innovation, accountability, and high performance. And it doesn't just benefit the team — it shows up in patient care too. When morale is strong and the team is united by a sense of purpose, the quality of care naturally improves. Patients can feel the difference when a team is functioning well — when people communicate clearly, support each other under pressure, and are emotionally present in the room. That's when the work becomes more than just a job — it becomes a shared mission. Team members feel inspired to bring their best — not just for the sake of performance, but because they're part of something that matters. When your team is thriving, your patients thrive too.

5.10 Fostering Diversity and Inclusion Through EQ

"It is not our differences that divide us. It is our inability to recognise, accept, and celebrate those differences."

— Audre Lorde

The diversity within our teams isn't just a box to tick — it's a strength. Our workplaces bring together people from a wide range of backgrounds, cultures, ages, belief systems, communication styles, and life experiences. And that variety doesn't just mirror the patients we serve — it enhances our ability to serve them well. But for that diversity to truly work in our favour, we need emotional intelligence. EQ helps us engage with those differences not with discomfort or defensiveness, but with curiosity, humility, and respect.

When a team is emotionally aware, diversity becomes a source of insight, creativity, and connection. Different perspectives challenge us to think differently, to see blind spots we might have missed, and to approach patient care from angles we wouldn't have considered alone. Emotional intelligence becomes the common language that helps us bridge those differences, so we can collaborate with empathy and confidence.

ADDRESSING UNCONSCIOUS BIAS

Of course, working in diverse teams also means facing some uncomfortable truths — including the fact that we all carry unconscious biases. These aren't always malicious or intentional — they're often automatic, deeply ingrained patterns shaped by our upbringing, social conditioning, and personal experiences. But just because they're subconscious doesn't mean they aren't doing harm. Unchecked, they can quietly undermine trust, stifle collaboration, and limit the potential of your team.

That's where EQ comes in. Self-awareness helps us spot those mental shortcuts and pause before we act on them. For instance, if you find yourself always assigning the more technical tasks to certain team members, it's worth asking why. Is it based on merit and skill — or an assumption? Similarly, if you notice a colleague's feedback bothering you more than others', take a moment to ask yourself whether it's the message — or the person delivering it — that's triggering a reaction.

THE LINK BETWEEN CULTURAL COMPETENCE AND EQ

Cultural competence is more than just being aware that people have different customs or holidays. It's about recognising how culture shapes beliefs, values, communication, and even how people experience health, illness, and care. It takes humility to acknowledge we don't know everything and empathy to hold space for perspectives that differ from our own.

You might have a patient who doesn't make direct eye contact, or a colleague who prefers indirect communication. These aren't flaws or failings — they're culturally informed behaviours. Emotional intelligence helps us meet people where they are rather than expecting them to adapt to us. When we're emotionally aware, we're less likely to judge and more likely to ask questions, listen with curiosity, and adapt our approach with respect.

BUILDING AN INCLUSIVE TEAM ENVIRONMENT

Creating an inclusive culture isn't a one-off initiative — it's an everyday practice. It starts with leaders, yes — but it's reinforced in every hallway conversation, every team huddle, and every decision made. Inclusion is about more than having diverse people on the team; it's about ensuring every voice is truly valued.

In my own practice, I've been lucky to work with a wonderfully diverse team — from different cultural, religious, and linguistic backgrounds. Over the years, I've learned so much just by being curious and open. I love hearing about their food, traditions, festivals, and family stories. It's not just fascinating — it deepens our connection and strengthens our team spirit. And practically speaking, it helps us better understand and relate to patients who share similar cultural backgrounds. When we understand where someone is coming from, we're much more likely to communicate with empathy and build trust.

That sense of connection shows up in the small, everyday moments too. Noticing when someone seems off and checking in. Giving quieter team members space to speak in meetings. Gently addressing dismissive or exclusive behaviour — even if it's subtle. Microaggressions, left unaddressed, erode trust over time. But when we address them kindly and directly, it sends a clear message: this is a place where everyone is safe, respected, and supported.

I try to lead by example in my clinic — whether that's making space for people to share feedback, revisiting decisions when someone raises a concern, or even just admitting when I've made a mistake. It's not about being perfect; it's about being approachable and fair. When we show people that they matter — not just for what they do, but for who they are — we create a team culture people want to be part of.

TRANSFORMING DIVERSITY INTO STRENGTH

Diversity can bring challenge and complexity — but it also brings depth, adaptability, and strength. When we pair it with emotional intelligence, it becomes a powerful asset. A team made up of people who think differently, solve problems differently, and bring unique life experiences to the table is a team that's more resilient, more innovative, and more equipped to meet the diverse needs of our patients.

It's like turning a kaleidoscope: each twist reveals a new pattern, a new way of seeing. And the more we practice engaging with difference — with openness, empathy, and a willingness to learn — the more beautiful that picture becomes. At the end of the day, this isn't about managing diversity — it's about celebrating it. It's about creating a workplace where people feel truly welcomed.

5.11 Feedback that Fuels Growth: Building Trust and Capability

---

> *"We all need people who will give us feedback. That's how we improve."*
>
> — Bill Gates

FEEDBACK AS A TOOL FOR EMOTIONAL AND PROFESSIONAL GROWTH

Feedback isn't just a formality or something to nervously save for a performance review — it's one of the most powerful tools we have for growth, learning, and building stronger teams. I've always liked the saying "failure is feedback" because it shifts the narrative away from blame and toward improvement. Feedback is knowledge, and knowledge is power. When feedback is a regular part of the culture — not something we only do when something's gone wrong — it becomes something people welcome rather than fear. In high-pressure moments, clear and concise communication becomes even more essential — both to avoid misunderstandings and to help the team stay aligned in the moment.

Emotionally intelligent feedback takes into account *how* the message is delivered — tone, timing, body language, and emotional readiness all matter just as much as the words themselves. If someone's just had a really rough day, it might not be the time to dissect everything that went wrong. But circle back at the right time, and that same feedback can land in a way that feels supportive rather than critical.

It's also about the language we use. Saying, "You handled that situation poorly," is likely to shut someone down. But reframing it with curiosity and care — "It looked like that situation didn't go quite as expected. Let's unpack what happened and figure out what we could try differently next time" — creates a safe space for learning. It moves the conversation from judgement to reflection, and that's where real growth happens.

In my own practice, I try to model this by checking in after challenging interactions or procedures. Rather than launching into a breakdown of what should've been done differently, I might ask, "How did you feel that went?" or "Is there anything you would change next time?" It opens the door to a two-way conversation — one that encourages self-awareness and creates space for honest dialogue. I want the other person to feel safe enough to unpack what happened and start exploring their own solutions, rather than waiting for me to spell it out for them. If I notice they're on the wrong track, or if there's something valuable that I've learned from my own past mistakes, I'll offer that perspective. But my goal isn't to lecture — it's to support. I want them to feel empowered, not corrected; like they're being coached, not critiqued.

And just as importantly, feedback should be two-sided. As leaders, we need to be open to hearing it too. That means creating an environment where team members feel safe to speak up — not just about systems or processes, but even about how we lead. I try to make it clear to my team that their insights and experiences matter just as much as mine. If something I've done has caused confusion, or if there's a better way I could support them, I want to know. The goal isn't to be perfect — it's to get better together. That takes humility, vulnerability, and a genuine willingness to listen without getting defensive. When we model that kind of openness ourselves, it signals to the team that feedback isn't a one-way street — it's a shared tool for growth, trust, and continuous improvement.

CONNECT BEFORE YOU CORRECT

One of the most powerful principles of effective feedback is this: connect before you correct. Before diving into what went wrong or what could've been done differently, take a moment to acknowledge the person's effort or intention. This isn't just about softening the blow — it's about creating a foundation of trust. When someone feels seen and appreciated, they're much more likely to stay open to hearing feedback and act on it.

For instance, you might say, "I know how much you care about the patient experience, and I really appreciate the time you spent with them." Once that connection is established, then move into the area that needs improvement — framed with the intention to support, not to criticise. When feedback comes from a place of shared purpose, it feels like a conversation, not a confrontation.

And it's not just *what* you say — it's *how* you say it. That is, it's not only the content — it's the context and tone that matter. Everything we say can be framed positively or negatively, and the difference can completely change how it's received. One of the most common mistakes I see is telling people what *not* to do. "Don't rush." "Don't forget to check the notes." "Don't stand like that." But here's the thing — our brains don't process negatives very well. Telling someone what not to do doesn't show them the path to get it right.

Instead, be specific about the behaviour you're aiming for:

Try, "Take your time with this part — accuracy matters more than speed," or "Make sure to check the patient notes before you call them in, so you're prepared." Clear, positive direction gives people something to work toward, not just something to avoid.

We've touched on this before, but it's worth repeating because it makes such a big difference: be mindful of how you transition between acknowledging someone's efforts and offering feedback. That tiny word — but — can completely unravel the goodwill you've just built. Saying something like, "I know you did your best, *but...*" often lands as dismissive, even if your intentions are good. Instead, swap it for "and". This small shift helps maintain connection and keeps the conversation constructive. For example, "I know you care deeply about your work, *and* I think there's an opportunity here to make it even better." It keeps the focus on growth without negating the effort already made.

It's these subtle shifts — connecting first, speaking with intention, and being clear about expectations — that turn feedback into fuel for growth, not a source of shame or stress.

CREATING EFFECTIVE FEEDBACK LOOPS

In a field like healthcare, where collaboration is everything, feedback is the thread that holds teams together. But feedback shouldn't be a one-off conversation — it needs to be an ongoing, two-way exchange. The most effective feedback loops thrive in environments built on trust and psychological safety — where people feel comfortable speaking up and confident that their voice will be met with curiosity rather than criticism. When feedback becomes a normal part of team culture, it strengthens relationships, promotes growth, and ultimately enhances patient care.

One way to build these feedback loops into your practice is by scheduling regular, dedicated feedback sessions. These can be short and informal, like a weekly check-in or a monthly team debrief. What matters is consistency. When feedback becomes a routine part of your team rhythm, it's no longer something to fear — it's something to expect and value. It also helps move feedback from reactive to proactive, shifting the focus from blame to learning.

Another powerful approach is peer-to-peer feedback. Encouraging team members to share insights with one another — not just with leadership — reinforces the idea that everyone has something to contribute and something to learn. This mutual exchange builds respect, accountability, and a sense of shared ownership over team performance. It also helps ease the pressure on leaders to be the sole source of guidance.

I remember an associate dentist once coming to me after a procedure, concerned about a possible infection control breach they'd noticed involving one of the dental assistants. While I appreciated them bringing it to me — and assured them I would address it — I gently encouraged them to speak directly with the assistant next time, in the moment. Not in a confrontational way, but with care, professionalism, and a mindset of shared responsibility. When team members feel safe and supported to offer each other feedback directly, it strengthens the culture of accountability and helps issues get addressed before they escalate or repeat. It also builds confidence and leadership capacity across the whole team, which is a win for everyone.

Another example from my clinic involved a small moment that had a big impact. Our practice manager had noticed that our new, younger receptionist was using very casual language when communicating with patients — both over the phone and in written communication. While the intent was friendly, phrases like "No worries" or "Yeah, that should be fine" lacked the clarity and professionalism we aim for in our practice. But instead of coming straight to me, the practice manager chose to address it directly with her in the moment, in a calm and respectful way.

She framed it with care: "You're doing a great job building rapport with patients, and I can tell they feel comfortable with you. One thing I've learned over the years is that in healthcare, the words we use really matter. Phrases that sound casual to us can sometimes come across as vague or even dismissive to patients. Let's workshop a few more polished ways to say the same thing so you're feeling confident and clear."

That conversation did more than correct the behaviour — it built trust. Our receptionist appreciated the feedback and didn't feel embarrassed or attacked. She made changes immediately and even started asking for input more proactively, which showed how empowered she felt by the interaction. It also reinforced to the team that feedback doesn't have to come from "above" — it can come from a place of mutual respect and shared standards.

Timely, real-time feedback is therefore also key. Waiting days or weeks to bring something up often means the moment (and the lesson) is lost. Addressing an issue right away — or soon after — keeps the context fresh and the insight clear, making the conversation far more meaningful. And importantly, feedback shouldn't only be about flagging what went wrong. A culture of feedback thrives when we're just as quick to acknowledge what's going right. Positive reinforcement not only boosts morale — it reinforces the behaviours and standards we want to see more of.

I also make it a point to remind my team that when I give feedback, I say what needs to be said, and then I move on. I don't believe in holding grudges or revisiting past mistakes through passive-aggressive comments. My very first boss had a habit of bringing up small missteps — even weeks or months later — under the guise of a joke. At first, I laughed along, but over time it chipped away at my confidence. It felt demeaning and left me walking on eggshells. That experience stuck with me and shaped the kind of leader I want to be: someone who supports growth, not someone who clings to past mistakes. Feedback should be honest, clear, and then left in the past — because we're all learning, and we deserve the opportunity to move forward.

When feedback is woven into everyday workflows — rather than being reserved for annual reviews or crisis moments — it sends a clear message: growth is ongoing, and everyone has a role in shaping the team's success. Feedback doesn't have to be formal or intimidating — it just needs to be regular, specific, and grounded in care.

THE ROLE OF STRUCTURED COMMUNICATION TOOLS

While emotionally intelligent conversations are essential, structure matters too. Tools like handoff protocols, checklists, communication boards, and team debriefs help ensure that vital information doesn't fall through the cracks — especially in high-pressure environments where stress can cloud memory or clarity. These systems bring order and consistency to communication, offering a dependable framework even when emotions are running high or time is limited.

Structured tools don't replace human connection — they enhance it. When used well, they support emotionally intelligent feedback by providing a shared language and expectations, reducing ambiguity, and helping teams stay aligned. For example, a well-run debrief after a challenging case allows space for reflection, shared learning, and improvement, rather than blame or speculation. Likewise, a clear handoff protocol ensures that key details are passed on, supporting both patient safety and team confidence. When structure and emotional awareness go hand in hand, communication becomes not only more effective, but more compassionate and empowering too.

NAVIGATING THE EMOTIONAL ASPECTS OF GIVING AND RECEIVING FEEDBACK

Giving and receiving feedback is rarely just about performance — it's emotional, and that's something we can't ignore. Whether you're offering feedback or on the receiving end of it, emotions are almost always in play. That's why emotional intelligence is essential. It helps us navigate these conversations with empathy, openness, and grace. When emotions run high — especially in the middle of a stressful shift — being able to stay composed and regulate your response allows you to lead with calm, not chaos. It also helps others feel safe enough to stay open to feedback or conversation, rather than shutting down.

For the person giving feedback, the challenge is balancing honesty with care. Your words should be clear and helpful, but they should also show that you genuinely want the other person to succeed. That means focusing on growth — not blame. For instance, if a team member struggled during a high-pressure moment, you might say, "I could see that was a really tough situation, and I want to help you feel more confident if something similar comes up again. Let's break it down together and figure out what we can learn from it." This kind of approach opens the door to reflection, not defensiveness.

On the receiving side, feedback can feel confronting — especially when it touches a nerve or hits an area where we already feel unsure of ourselves. That's totally human. Feedback can stir up defensiveness, embarrassment, or even shame. But the way we process those emotions makes all the difference. Developing the self-awareness to recognise when we're feeling triggered — and then pausing before reacting — can transform feedback into something empowering rather than painful.

I try to advise my team that feedback is a gift. It's not always wrapped in a pretty bow, but it's offered with the intent to help you grow. When we start to see it that way, it becomes less personal and more purposeful. That shift in mindset — seeing feedback as insight, not insult — takes emotional regulation, especially in the heat of the moment. Sometimes it's as simple as taking a deep breath, really listening, and reminding yourself not to jump to conclusions. Give yourself the space to respond, not react.

A powerful way to engage with feedback is by asking thoughtful follow-up questions. Things like, "Could you give me a specific example?" or "What would doing this differently look like next time?" These questions show that you're not only open to the feedback — you're curious and committed to learning from it. And they help clarify expectations, which is just as important as the feedback itself.

Ultimately, receiving feedback well is an act of self-awareness and humility. It means putting your ego aside, recognising that none of us are finished products, and embracing the sometimes uncomfortable process of becoming better. The most respected people I've worked with aren't the ones who do everything perfectly — they're the ones who take feedback on board with grace and use it to grow. One of the things I admire most about my new graduate associate is her willingness to do exactly that. She listens openly, reflects thoughtfully, and genuinely wants to improve. That attitude is one of the key reasons I was happy to offer her a role and invest the time to mentor her over hiring a more experienced dentist — because skill can be taught, but mindset is everything.

FEEDBACK IN ACTION: THE TRUST APPROACH

The ability to give feedback with empathy, clarity, and purpose is essential — not just for individual growth, but for building a culture of accountability, trust, and continual improvement. One of the most helpful ways I've found to remember how to deliver feedback well is through the acronym TRUST. It captures the five key principles that can guide your approach, whether you're offering praise, addressing a concern, or helping someone grow in their role.

T – Timely

Feedback loses its impact the longer we wait. Aim to give feedback as soon as possible — ideally in the moment or within 24–48 hours — while the situation is still fresh in everyone's mind. Whether you're acknowledging something done well or addressing a mistake, prompt feedback keeps the message clear, specific, and actionable. This allows team members to apply corrections or insights right away, thereby reducing the risk of recurring errors. For instance, if a nurse improperly documents a patient's chart, discussing it during the same shift ensures the incident is fresh in their memory.

In my practice, I make it a point to let my team know that if something needs to be addressed, I'll do it straight away — and once we've had the conversation, it's done. We move on. I won't bring it up weeks later or joke about it in passing. As I mentioned earlier, my first boss used to do that all the time, and it always left me feeling uneasy, like I was being quietly judged. That's not the kind of culture I want to create. Timely feedback allows us to deal with issues while they're small, fix them together, and get back to doing what we do best — taking great care of our patients.

R – Right Person

Before giving feedback, ask yourself: Am I the best person to have this conversation? Sometimes, someone else may have more context, a stronger rapport, or greater expertise in the area being addressed — and that can make all the difference in how the feedback is received. This isn't about avoiding difficult conversations; it's about making sure the message is delivered with the greatest possible clarity and impact.

For example, if a junior doctor makes a prescribing error, it might be tempting for a colleague to step in and address it immediately. But depending on the relationship dynamics and the complexity of the issue, it may be more appropriate for their supervising physician to step in instead. That leader not only has the clinical authority but also the mentorship role to frame the conversation in a way that fosters learning without undermining confidence.

Of course, this doesn't mean brushing things under the rug or saying "That's not my job." If you're not the right person to deliver the feedback directly, you can still ensure it's addressed by tactfully flagging it to someone who is. The key is to do this without gossip or blame — always with professionalism and the shared goal of high-quality care. This thoughtful approach maintains trust, protects relationships, and ensures that feedback lands in the most meaningful way.

U – Understand

Before you correct someone, seek first to understand their perspective. Emotional intelligence plays a big role here. Get curious about why something happened, and don't assume intent. Ask open-ended questions, acknowledge effort, and give the other person a chance to share their side. When people feel heard and understood, they're far more open to hearing what you have to say.

It's also worth remembering that when we feel heard, something shifts internally. That pent-up stress or tension starts to release, and suddenly the mind becomes more open to problem-solving. We shift from feeling attacked to feeling supported — which is where real growth happens.

S – Speak Face-to-Face

Whenever possible, deliver feedback in person. Written messages, even when well-intentioned, can be misinterpreted. There's just no substitute for face-to-face connection. Your tone of voice, body language, and eye contact all help convey warmth and respect — especially when the topic is sensitive.

Sitting down with a colleague in a private setting conveys respect and attentiveness, ensuring the message is received in the spirit it's intended. That said, "face-to-face" doesn't mean formal or intimidating. Sometimes it's a quick chat in the break room or a quiet word after a procedure. A supportive, real-time conversation is almost always better than an email or a message left to simmer. What matters most is the tone and intention behind it.

T – Think Objectively

Keep the focus on the behaviour, not the person. Objective, specific feedback prevents the other person from feeling judged or attacked. Instead of saying, "You're disorganised," try, "The chart wasn't updated in time, which caused some delays for the next appointment. Let's look at what happened and figure out how to avoid that next time." Stick to the facts as much as possible.

The goal is to be constructive, not critical. Let the person know you believe in their ability to do better and that you're here to help them succeed. You can also personalise the feedback with your own experiences — for example, "I used to struggle with this too when I first started. What helped me was..." These moments of shared vulnerability build trust and connection while keeping the conversation growth-focused.

WHY TRUST WORKS

When we deliver feedback using these principles, we reinforce the emotional safety and mutual respect that make high-performing teams possible. Feedback no longer feels like a confrontation — it feels like a collaboration. And when your team knows they can trust you to be fair, clear, and constructive, they're far more likely to listen, learn, and grow. In the end, feedback isn't about pointing out what's wrong — it's about nurturing what's possible.

Chapter 6

Patient Trust: Safe, Seen and Supported

6.1 Building Patient Trust from the First Encounter

"To be trusted is a greater compliment than being loved."

— George MacDonald

Trust is the foundation of every meaningful patient relationship — a bridge that takes time to build, yet can be shaken in a moment. And it doesn't begin with the treatment plan — it begins with the welcome, the warmth, and the way we show up.

Imagine a patient walking into your clinic, nervous and unsure. Before any words are exchanged, they're met with a warm smile, open body language, and a calm, kind tone. That moment says, "You're safe here. I've got you." These seemingly small gestures are actually the building blocks of trust — and they all stem from emotional intelligence. When we tune in to how our patients are feeling and respond with presence and empathy, we make space for connection and safety from the very beginning.

THE TRUST TRIANGLE

The dynamics of trust in both patient and team relationships can be visualised through the Trust Triangle, made up of three key elements:

- Transparency and Honesty
- Consistency in Care
- Owning Mistakes with Integrity

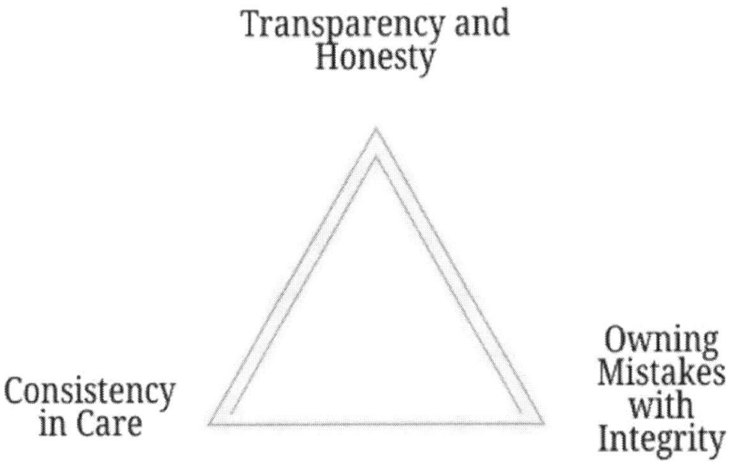

Each point reinforces the others. We can't be consistent if we're not honest. We can't own mistakes without vulnerability. And we can't be transparent if we're unwilling to do the emotional work of empathy and self-awareness. Trust isn't something we have; it's something we earn — one interaction, one small gesture, at a time.

TRANSPARENCY AND HONESTY

Trust isn't built on kindness alone — it's built through emotional intelligence in action. That includes transparency and honesty, especially when we're delivering difficult news or outlining treatment options. We don't always need to have all the answers — but we do need the courage to say, "I'm not sure, but I'll find out." It shows patients that we respect their autonomy and want to partner with them in their care — not just tell them what to do. This kind of candour doesn't undermine our credibility; it strengthens it. It shows patients that we're not here to pretend we're perfect. We're a team in their care and will always act in their best interest.

CONSISTENCY IN CARE

Trust doesn't come from one good appointment — it comes from showing up the same way, every time. Whether it's a routine clean or a difficult extraction, patients want to know that we'll be patient when they're anxious, clear when they're confused, and compassionate no matter how hectic the day gets. Consistency sends a message: I care about you.

And this consistency doesn't just apply to the clinician — it applies to the entire team. Patients may not see the full picture behind the scenes, but they feel its effects. What patients feel in the chair is a direct reflection of what's happening behind the scenes. When they see a team that communicates well, supports each other, and genuinely enjoys working together, they feel more relaxed, confident, and cared for. What happens inside the team is felt by those outside it.

THE FOLLOW-UP: EXTENDING CARE BEYOND THE APPOINTMENT

One of the simplest but most powerful ways to build trust is through follow-up care. After delivering unsettling news or completing a difficult procedure, a follow-up call the next day can make all the difference. It gives patients space to ask questions they may have forgotten during the appointment, reassures them that their care doesn't end the moment they walk out the door and reinforces that they're not alone in their care journey. It tells them, you still matter to us.

In my practice, we make it a priority to follow up after any challenging procedure — whether it's a wisdom tooth extraction, a root canal, or a particularly uncomfortable appointment. A quick phone call to check on how the patient is doing helps ease their anxiety, reassures them that what they're feeling is normal, and gives us a chance to address any concerns early. It also offers a chance to humanise the experience — to remind them that behind the treatment, there's someone who genuinely cares about how they're feeling.

But it's about more than clinical care — it's about emotional reassurance. These small gestures often make a lasting impression, and I've found they go a long way in building long-term relationships with patients. When people feel cared for on a personal level, they become more understanding and forgiving if something doesn't go exactly as planned. Trust becomes the cushion that softens those moments, allowing us to navigate them together with empathy and transparency.

OWNING MISTAKES WITH INTEGRITY

We all make mistakes. What matters most is how we handle them. I've learned that when something goes wrong, honesty paired with empathy can actually deepen trust rather than damage it. Patients don't expect perfection — they expect accountability. A calm explanation, a sincere apology, and a plan to make it right can turn a moment of disappointment into a foundation for long-term trust. It shows that we're human — and that we care.

I'll never forget one patient who came to see me while transitioning from a finance career to becoming a school teacher. She was excited but anxious — especially about how her students might perceive her smile. We started with some fillings and whitening, and eventually placed two new crowns on her front teeth. The day they went in, she was absolutely over the moon — smiling and glowing with confidence.

But later that evening, she went home and her young daughter, with all the innocent honesty of a child, told her she looked like a rabbit. The comment devastated her. She spent the whole weekend crying and feeling self-conscious. First thing Monday morning, she called me in tears. I listened, reassured her, and told her without hesitation that I'd be happy to redo her crowns. All I want is for my patients to be happy with their smiles — and to feel confident in them.

We redid the crowns, and she now absolutely loves them. The trust we had built meant she felt comfortable enough to come to me with her distress — and trusted me to make it right. And I did, because that's what matters. That kind of integrity doesn't just resolve a concern — it strengthens the relationship and creates lasting confidence in every interaction that follows.

Trust becomes the cushion that softens those moments, allowing us to navigate them together with empathy and transparency.

6.2 Managing Expectations with Clarity and Compassion

> *"If you align expectations with reality, you will never be disappointed."*
>
> — Terrell Owens

In healthcare, where every interaction holds the weight of hope and uncertainty, managing patient expectations is both an art and a responsibility. Patients don't just bring us symptoms — they bring stories, past experiences, fears, and dreams. It's our role to navigate these emotional landscapes with empathy, ensuring their understanding of treatment possibilities aligns with reality. This delicate balance requires more than clinical knowledge — it calls for emotional intelligence.

MEETING PATIENTS WHERE THEY ARE

To build trust, we must meet patients on their level — not from a place of superiority, but from one of partnership. We may hold specialised knowledge, but that doesn't make us more important. When we communicate using plain language, we're not dumbing things down — we're demonstrating respect. It reassures patients that they're included in the process and that we're working together toward their health goals.

I've found analogies especially helpful when explaining complex conditions. For example, when discussing gum disease, I often compare it to termites silently eating away at the foundation of a house. That imagery helps patients understand the seriousness of the condition and why addressing it is so important. Similarly, I sometimes describe enamel erosion like a worn-down road surface — gradually thinned by constant wear, leaving the tooth more vulnerable to damage. These kinds of comparisons bridge the gap between medical terminology and lived experience, empowering patients with the clarity they need to take meaningful action.

BALANCING HOPE WITH REALITY

Setting realistic expectations is a tightrope act — one that requires empathy, emotional awareness, and strong communication. Patients bring more than just questions; they bring anxiety, uncertainty, and a deep desire for reassurance. If we respond too clinically, we risk sounding cold or dismissive. But if we avoid the hard truths, we risk fostering false hope. By listening actively and validating their concerns, we can frame discussions around treatment possibilities and limitations in a way that's both honest and compassionate.

Emotional intelligence allows us to approach these conversations with compassion. Instead of a blunt "This can't be fixed," we might say, "Here's what we can do, and here's what the limitations are." It's about preserving dignity while being truthful. Engaging patients in an honest, two-way dialogue helps them feel informed and supported, even when the news is difficult.

I remember a patient who came into the clinic deeply distressed after breaking one of his front teeth off clean at the gum line. It had previously been restored with a post and crown, but now the root was fractured and unsalvageable. Clinically, there was no doubt — it needed to be extracted and replaced. But emotionally, the patient couldn't accept it. He kept pleading with us to just glue the tooth back in, desperate for a simple fix. In that moment, it wasn't about logic — it was about fear, shock, and loss.

We had to meet him where he was. Instead of dismissing his request, we acknowledged his distress and gently explained why reattaching the tooth wasn't possible. We shifted the focus toward what was possible — outlining his options and reassuring him that we would support him every step of the way. That conversation wasn't easy, but it was necessary. And because it was handled with empathy and grace, it became a turning point — transforming fear into understanding and helplessness into trust.

In the end, he chose to replace the tooth with a dental implant. He was not only thrilled with the final outcome but deeply appreciative of the care and understanding he received during such an upsetting time. That trust, built in a moment of vulnerability, became the foundation for an ongoing relationship marked by confidence, collaboration, and mutual respect.

NAVIGATING DISAPPOINTMENT

Despite our best efforts, there are times when things don't go as hoped. A patient may feel frustrated, disheartened, or even angry — and those responses are completely valid. In these moments, emotional intelligence becomes essential. We must hold space for these emotions without rushing to fix them. Acknowledging their disappointment with statements like, "I can see why this would be so frustrating for you," can have a profound impact. It shows them they're not alone in their experience.

But it doesn't stop there — our role is also to help guide them forward. That might mean reframing expectations, offering alternatives, or simply being a calm, caring presence as they process.

One of the most effective ways to ease future disappointment is by setting clear expectations from the very beginning. When we outline all reasonable possibilities — including the less desirable ones — we create emotional preparedness. It's not about being pessimistic; it's about being transparent. If we don't set these expectations early, and something goes wrong, any explanation risks sounding like an excuse. But when patients have been gently and clearly informed of potential complications from the outset, they may still feel disappointed — but they're far less likely to feel blindsided.

I once had a patient who came in with what appeared to be a moderate cavity in a back molar. Based on the initial exam and x-rays, we believed it could be resolved with a straightforward filling. Before beginning though, I explained that there was a chance the decay might be deeper than expected — and if it was, we might need to consider a root canal and crown to save the tooth or extraction. The patient understood and was hopeful that it wouldn't come to that.

Unfortunately, once I began removing the decay, I could see the damage was far more extensive than anticipated. The nerve had likely been compromised. I paused, re-explained the situation, and outlined the new treatment options. The patient was understandably disappointed — but because we'd discussed this possibility ahead of time, they already had a framework to process the change in plan. They didn't feel like it was a bait-and-switch. They felt informed, respected, and supported.

These moments require emotional awareness and sensitivity. They remind us that patient care is never just about procedures — it's about people, expectations, and how we show up for them when plans need to change. I didn't launch straight into the technical details or pressure them into a decision. I acknowledged the disappointment and said, "I know this isn't what you were hoping to hear today, and I'm really sorry. I'll support you with whatever decision you make, and we'll take the next step together." That shift — from clinical problem-solver to compassionate partner — helped restore calm and trust.

These situations are never easy, but when handled with presence and empathy, they can strengthen the therapeutic relationship. Disappointment is part of healthcare — but so is the opportunity to walk patients through it with care and understanding.

Managing expectations isn't about softening the truth or steering the conversation — it's about creating a partnership built on honesty, trust, and mutual respect. Patients shouldn't feel like passengers in their own care. With emotional intelligence, we can create an alliance where both voices matter.

In this kind of therapeutic relationship, our clinical expertise and the patient's lived experience come together to shape a realistic and hopeful treatment plan. When we get that balance right — when patients feel seen, informed, and empowered — their overall experience is improved, even when outcomes don't match initial hopes.

At its heart, managing expectations with clarity and compassion is about honouring both the science and the story. And when we do that well, we don't just provide care — we build lasting trust.

6.3 Breaking Bad News with Emotional Awareness

"Sometimes it takes only one act of kindness and caring to change a person's life."

— Jackie Chan

Delivering bad news is one of the most emotionally charged tasks in healthcare. These moments carry immense weight, shaping our relationships with patients and leaving lasting impressions. While clinical detachment has its place, difficult conversations call for presence, empathy, and emotional intelligence.

PREPARING FOR THE CONVERSATION

Before walking into the room to deliver bad news, it's crucial to prepare — not just in terms of facts, but also emotionally and mentally. Grounding yourself emotionally helps you show up with presence and clarity. Bad news is rarely just medical; it's personal, often life-changing. It can stir grief, fear, anger, or hopelessness. By entering these conversations with a sense of presence and care, we can offer more than just information — we can offer a steadying hand in what is often an overwhelming moment.

One scenario that stands out in my practice involved a patient who desperately wanted to save a back tooth that had cracked all the way through. Despite their wishes, there was no viable option but extraction. For many, losing a tooth might not seem like "bad news" on the scale of life-altering diagnoses. But for this patient, the news was deeply distressing — a reminder of past dental trauma and a fear of further loss. I knew this news had to be handled delicately. I sat down, made eye contact, and calmly explained the situation in terms they could relate to, using an analogy about a foundation that can no longer support its structure. I validated their feelings and reassured them we'd create a treatment plan that restored both function and confidence. Their trust in me hinged on how I approached that moment, and I've never forgotten how significant it was for them.

BALANCING EMPATHY AND PROFESSIONALISM

Delivering bad news isn't just about what you say; it's about how you say it. Patients don't just need honesty — they need humanity. Striking the right balance means softening your tone, allowing silence, and staying present as emotions unfold. It's about actively listening, being attuned to the emotions of the patient and their family and creating space for their reactions. These moments often demand more silence than speech — giving patients the chance to absorb the news, ask questions, or simply express their feelings in a safe space. When handled with grace, these interactions can be transformative.

On the other hand, the absence of empathy can turn an already difficult situation into something truly harrowing. Not long ago, a dear friend's mum was transferred to palliative care after a long and courageous battle with cancer. This was an incredibly distressing time for their family, but the compassion shown by the palliative care nurses provided comfort amidst the grief. They treated her with such care and dignity, and their empathy helped the family feel supported.

Unfortunately, the same couldn't be said for the doctors who came through to check on her. Time and again, they asked bluntly, "Where do you want to die — here or at home?" with little sensitivity to the emotional context. To the family, those words cut deeper than the diagnosis itself. It's a stark reminder that how we deliver difficult news matters as much as the message itself. These interactions should be approached with grace, care, and a deep respect for the person and their loved ones.

Reflection: Holding Space While Speaking Truth

Delivering difficult news is never easy — but it's often defining. These are the moments patients remember. They shape how safe someone feels in your care and how deeply they trust your judgment and compassion.

Take a moment to reflect on one of these conversations in your own career. This isn't about getting it perfect — it's about understanding your emotional response, your communication choices, and your growth as a clinician and human being.

- *How did it feel — for you and for the patient?*
- *What helped you navigate it well?*
- *What would you do differently next time?*
- *How do you want patients to feel after receiving difficult news from you?*

SUPPORTING PATIENTS AFTER THE NEWS

The emotional work doesn't end once the news is delivered. Patients and families often need time and support to process what they've just heard. Following up, offering a second appointment to address additional concerns, providing resources for emotional or practical support or simply being present — all of this reassures patients that their care matters beyond the moment.

A follow-up call, especially after a difficult procedure or consultation, can make a world of difference. It's a small gesture, but it reassures patients that we see them as individuals, not just cases. After a particularly challenging extraction or procedure, I make it a point to check in with patients the next day. It lets them know that their comfort and recovery matter to me, and it often opens the door for questions or concerns they didn't think of previously.

CARING FOR OURSELVES, TOO

Delivering bad news doesn't just affect the person receiving it — it affects the person delivering it, too. As healthcare professionals, we are trained to hold space for others, to stay composed, and to keep moving forward. But that doesn't mean we're immune to the emotional weight of these conversations. In fact, the more connected and compassionate we are, the more likely we are to carry that weight with us.

It's easy to underestimate how these moments accumulate. One difficult conversation might feel manageable, but over time — especially without a way to process — it can lead to emotional exhaustion or even burnout. That's why it's so important to intentionally build in practices that help us release and reflect, rather than absorb and store.

Sometimes, that means a debrief with a trusted colleague — someone who understands what it's like and can help you make sense of the emotional undercurrent. Other times, it's about creating private moments to pause: journaling about what happened, taking a few minutes to walk or breathe, or simply acknowledging to yourself, "That was hard." These small acts of emotional hygiene aren't indulgent — they're necessary. They help us stay grounded, resilient, and capable of showing up with compassion.

It's also important to recognise the power of peer support. Whether it's an informal chat in the tea room or a more structured reflection in team meetings, sharing the emotional load helps break the isolation that often comes with emotionally challenging work. When we normalise talking about how these moments affect us, we not only support ourselves — we create a safer, more supportive culture for everyone.

At its core, delivering bad news is about human connection. It asks us to sit with pain, uncertainty, and sometimes even despair — and to do so with grace. But we can't do that sustainably if we don't care for ourselves with the same empathy we offer others. Whether it's the loss of a tooth or the acceptance of terminal illness, these conversations shape the emotional landscape of our work. Honouring our own emotional response to them is not a weakness — it's a sign of strength, and of the deep humanity we bring to this profession.

6.4 Supporting Grieving Families with Empathy

"Only time and tears take away grief; that is what they are for."

— Terry Pratchett

In the quiet aftermath of loss — when the hospital monitors fall silent and the room shifts from urgency to stillness — our role as healthcare professionals changes. We move from clinical decision-makers to compassionate companions, holding space for those who are hurting.

Supporting grieving families is one of the most human, and humbling, responsibilities we carry. It goes beyond medical care — it's about showing up with presence, sensitivity, and emotional awareness.

UNDERSTANDING THE SHAPE OF GRIEF

Grief is not a one-size-fits-all experience. It's not linear or predictable. It's messy, complex, and deeply personal, presenting in countless ways for different people. Some might cry openly; others may withdraw or express anger. Our job is not to diagnose these reactions, but to honour them. Emotional intelligence helps us respond without judgment and tune into the emotional undercurrents that may not be spoken out loud.

This begins with active listening — being fully present to what is said, and what is not. I once heard a story from a physician friend who sat with a father who had just lost his teenage son. Instead of trying to say the "right" thing, the doctor simply listened. The father shifted between tears and laughter as he shared stories of his son. In that space, what mattered wasn't clinical expertise — it was presence. That story has stayed with me. It reminds me that in moments of raw loss, our ability to be quietly present can speak louder than any words and the importance of creating an environment where people feel safe and supported.

HONOURING CULTURAL AND SPIRITUAL TRADITIONS

Grief is shaped not just by emotion, but by culture. Different communities have unique ways of processing death, honouring the deceased, and supporting one another. These rituals may seem unfamiliar, but they carry deep meaning — and respecting them is a vital part of providing emotionally intelligent care. Sometimes, showing cultural sensitivity is as simple as asking, "What would be helpful for you right now?" or "Are there any traditions or customs you'd like us to support?" These small questions communicate deep respect and validate the family's experience.

A physician once shared an experience with me about caring for a patient whose family held deeply spiritual beliefs about the process of death. The family had specific rituals they wanted to perform at the bedside, and the care team ensured they had the space, privacy and time to carry them out. It wasn't just about honouring their cultural practices; it was about showing genuine care for their grieving process in a way that was meaningful to them. This story really highlighted the importance of respecting individual traditions and the profound impact it can have on the healing journey of those left behind.

EXTENDING CAFE BEYOND THE MOMENT

Grief doesn't end when the bed is emptied or the room is cleaned. While the intensity may ebb with time, the ache of loss often lingers. For families, the hardest days often come after the final goodbye. That's why long-term support matters. Follow-up calls, written notes, or even offering grief counselling referrals can be profoundly meaningful.

I've seen how much comfort a simple call can bring. A short check-in — "How are you doing?" or "We're still thinking of you" — reminds families that their loved one wasn't just a patient, and that their own grief still matters. It tells them: We see you. We remember.

CARING FOR OURSELVES, TOO

Providing comfort in the face of loss takes an emotional toll. We absorb the sadness of others, often without having the time or space to process our own reactions. Emotional fatigue is real — and if unacknowledged, it can lead to burnout or compassion fatigue.

That's why self-care must be part of this work. Whether it's debriefing with a colleague, stepping outside for a few quiet minutes, journaling, or seeking support through therapy or peer groups, these acts of emotional hygiene matter. They're not indulgences — they're safeguards. Caring for others means caring for ourselves, too.

HUMANITY IN GRIEF

Helping families through grief and loss is about being present in their pain, honouring their unique experiences, and offering a steady presence as they navigate an incredibly difficult journey. Emotional intelligence allows us to do this with sensitivity and authenticity, creating a space where families feel supported, respected, and cared for — even in their darkest moments. Through this approach, we can fulfil one of the greatest callings of our profession: to be a source of comfort and strength when it matters most.

6.5 Communicating Across Cultures and Language Barriers

> *"Good communication is the bridge between confusion and clarity."*
>
> — Nat Turner

Serving diverse communities means encountering a rich tapestry of cultures, languages, and perspectives. These differences present both challenges and opportunities — especially when cultural nuances or language gaps add complexity to communication. In these moments, emotional intelligence becomes essential, allowing us to connect with respect, compassion, and curiosity.

CULTURAL COMPETENCE AND RESPONSIVENESS

Cultural competence is the ability to be respectful and open toward different cultural perspectives. It involves learning about other cultures, avoiding assumptions, and building rapport across differences. But cultural responsiveness takes it further: it means actively adapting our care based on the unique cultural lens of the patient in front of us. It's not just about what we consider respectful — it's about what they perceive as respectful.

A cornerstone of this is self-determination. Culturally safe care is defined by the recipient, not the provider. As clinicians, we must regularly reflect on how our intentions are received and be willing to shift our approach in real-time. For instance, something as simple as how we greet a patient, touch their arm, or ask personal questions can be interpreted differently depending on their cultural background. Emotional intelligence helps us remain open, observant, and adaptable — allowing us to serve the person, not just the condition.

BUILDING A DIVERSE AND INCLUSIVE TEAM

To meet the needs of a diverse patient population, it helps to have a team that reflects that diversity. Hiring staff from various cultural and linguistic backgrounds doesn't just improve communication — it sends a powerful message to patients: You are welcome here. You are seen.

Representation matters. A patient who shares a language, cultural background, or life experience with a team member may feel more comfortable opening up, especially when navigating complex or vulnerable conversations. This kind of connection can build trust where words alone might fall short.

Inclusivity should also extend inward. Within the team, fostering open conversations about cultural identity, personal values, and different traditions enriches workplace culture. Whether it's celebrating religious holidays, learning greetings in another language, or respectfully exploring one another's worldviews, these moments of cultural exchange deepen connection and strengthen team cohesion.

CREATIVE COMMUNICATION STRATEGIES

Building rapport without relying solely on words requires creativity and emotional intelligence. Techniques like mirroring body language, maintaining eye contact to convey attentiveness, and using visual aids or drawings to explain medical concepts can be incredibly effective. You might also consider translated diagrams, or even gesture-based explanations to build shared understanding. These simple tools reduce anxiety and show that you're making an effort to include the patient fully in their care.

Using plain, accessible language is equally important. This doesn't mean talking down – it means stripping away medical jargon and connecting with clarity. Analogies can make abstract concepts relatable. As mentioned earlier, I often explain gum disease by comparing it to termites silently eating away at the foundation of a house. It's simple, vivid, and helps patients grasp the seriousness of the condition in a way that sticks.

Similarly, when talking about tooth loss, I might use a bookshelf analogy: "Imagine pulling one book out of a tightly packed shelf – the ones on either side can start to lean or fall. That's what happens when a tooth is lost – the neighbouring teeth can shift or topple, leading to alignment and bite problems." These everyday comparisons not only bridge the gap between medical complexity and patient understanding – they empower patients to make informed decisions about their care.

THE ROLE OF NON-VERBAL COMMUNICATION

When language barriers exist, non-verbal communication becomes a powerful bridge. A warm smile, a nod of reassurance, open and welcoming body language – these gestures are universally recognised and often carry more emotional weight than spoken words. They help put patients at ease, signalling respect, kindness, and a willingness to connect, even when vocabulary fails.

Simple actions — like sitting at eye level instead of standing over a patient, softening your facial expression, or keeping an open posture — communicate safety and attentiveness. Touch, too, when appropriate and culturally sensitive, can be incredibly grounding. A light hand on the shoulder or a supportive pat on the arm can say, "I'm here with you" in ways that words sometimes can't.

Likewise, being attuned to a patient's non-verbal cues — posture, facial expressions, restlessness, or even averted eye contact — can reveal discomfort, fear, or misunderstanding that might not be explicitly expressed. I once had a patient who barely spoke any English. While she nodded throughout our conversation, I noticed she clutched her handbag tightly and shifted nervously in her seat. Rather than assume she understood, I paused and gently said, "It's okay to ask questions," using slow speech and simple gestures. She immediately relaxed and motioned to her daughter sitting quietly in the corner to act as an interpreter, which changed the direction of the appointment for the better. That moment reminded me that true communication isn't always verbal — it's about noticing what isn't said and responding with care.

Adapting your tone, pace, or physical presence in response to these cues shows emotional intelligence in action. It demonstrates that you're not just focused on the task — you're focused on the person. And that effort to connect, even non-verbally, often speaks louder than anything we could say.

PARTNERING WITH INTERPRETERS

Professional interpreters are invaluable in overcoming language barriers, but how we engage with them can significantly shape the patient's experience. Before the conversation begins, take a moment to brief the interpreter — let them know if sensitive topics may arise or if there's specific medical language that will need clarification. This helps them prepare not just linguistically, but emotionally, too.

During the interaction, always speak directly to the patient — not the interpreter. Make eye contact, use the patient's name, and remain fully engaged. This preserves the relational aspect of care and reinforces the patient's sense of agency and dignity. After the consultation, consider debriefing with the interpreter to clarify any subtleties, especially if the discussion involved emotionally charged or complex information. It's important to ensure mutual understanding and clarify any subtleties that may have been missed.

That said, access to professional interpreters isn't always possible — particularly in time-pressured or resource-limited settings. In these situations, clinicians may rely on a trusted family member or friend of the patient to help with communication. While not ideal, this can sometimes be the most immediate and practical solution.

I was reminded of this recently when my grandmother was admitted to hospital. She speaks broken English and, although she's fiercely independent and eager to communicate with clinicians herself, she often misunderstands more than she realises. One day, a speech pathologist visited to assess her swallowing following concerns from nursing staff. The clinician did an excellent job — speaking slowly, using simple language and hand gestures — but my grandmother wasn't comprehending the questions clearly and wasn't communicating her answers accurately either. Fortunately, I happened to be there and was able to translate and advocate for her. Without that support, her care plan may have been based on incomplete or misunderstood information.

That moment deeply reinforced the importance of ensuring that communication is not only delivered clearly, but also understood and received accurately. When there is any doubt, we must pause and ask: is this truly a shared understanding? And if not, what support — whether a professional interpreter or a trusted companion — can help bridge the gap? In healthcare, misunderstandings can have real consequences, and it's our responsibility to ensure language never becomes a barrier to safe, compassionate care.

6.6 Emotional Intelligence in Vulnerable Care Settings: Long-Term Support and Paediatric Settings

> *"Too often we underestimate the power of a touch, a smile, a kind word... all of which have the potential to turn a life around."*
>
> — Leo Buscaglia

When caring for people at their most vulnerable — whether in long-term aged care or paediatric settings — emotional intelligence is essential. These environments require us to move beyond task-based care and step into a space of deeper connection, presence, and compassion. In both cases, the people we care for are often dependent on us — not just for clinical support, but for emotional safety, reassurance, and a sense of being known.

BUILDING RELATIONSHIPS THAT LAST

In long-term care settings, where clinicians may spend months or even years with residents, relationships are built slowly and meaningfully. Over time, these bonds often resemble family ties. You learn their stories — their favourite songs, the food they miss, the people they love. In return, you become a constant in their ever-changing world, a familiar face in a sea of unfamiliarity.

Before I became a dentist, I worked as a pharmacy assistant and often visited patients in long-term care homes. I still remember the joy that a small, familiar gesture could bring — taking a moment to chat, asking about a grandchild's visit, or remembering that someone preferred their tablets crushed with yoghurt. These weren't just courtesies — they were connections. And those moments taught me that in aged care, it's the emotional presence we bring, not just the medication we deliver, that makes the biggest difference.

Something as simple as remembering a resident's wedding anniversary or asking about their children can bring deep comfort. It shows that they are more than just patients — they are people with rich histories, personalities, and inner lives. These small, human touches contribute to a sense of dignity and belonging that improves not only emotional wellbeing but often physical health outcomes too.

Aged care can also bring up complex emotions — loneliness, grief, fear of decline. Recognising emotional shifts early — like withdrawal, increased irritability, or changes in behaviour — can prompt timely support. Whether that support involves social engagement, therapeutic activities, or simply sitting and listening, emotional presence can be just as powerful as clinical intervention.

COMMUNICATING WITH CHILDREN

In paediatric care, we see vulnerability through a different lens. Children may not yet have the vocabulary or emotional awareness to express how they feel — but that doesn't mean they aren't feeling deeply. This is where emotional intelligence becomes a bridge. Communicating with children means tuning into their world: using age-appropriate language, metaphors they understand, and non-verbal cues that make them feel safe.

When children come in for a dental visit, especially for the first time, it's often a whole production — and rightly so. We're laying the foundation for how they'll view oral healthcare for years to come. I firmly believe that we should never rush or push. Some children are comfortable from day one, while others need time to warm up. With some, we spend the first one or two appointments simply helping them feel at ease — talking, showing them around, or letting them watch a sibling in the chair.

Predictability and structure also play a key role in helping children feel safe. I try to keep the rhythm of the visit familiar — maybe starting with a friendly chat, then a ride in the chair, then counting teeth — so even if we don't get far in the first appointment, the experience is consistent. It's not about rushing. It's about building trust, appointment by appointment. If we push too soon, we risk cementing fear instead of trust. But if we take our time, they often surprise us with how much they're willing to try.

When explaining something to a child, I try to avoid medical jargon entirely. I'll say, "We're going to take some pictures of your teeth," instead of "Let's get an x-ray," or "Your tooth has a wobbly friend," rather than, "Your tooth is mobile and due to exfoliate soon." These changes might seem small, but they shift the tone from clinical to conversational, helping reduce fear and confusion. Sometimes I'll ask, "Can I count your teeth?" — a much less intimidating request than "Can I examine your mouth?" I use playful language that they can relate to. I might say, "Let's tickle your teeth today,", "Your teeth are going to have a little shower," or "This is Mr Sucky Straw — he's going to drink up all the water for you." These phrases help make unfamiliar tools and sensations less scary.

I often demonstrate everything on the back of their hand before we try it in their mouth. It gives them a sense of control and helps build trust. If I can't demonstrate it — for example, if it's a mirror or something less tactile — I'll show them instead, explaining what it looks like and how it works. I also always talk them through what to expect next, step by step, so there are no surprises. That way, they feel included in the process rather than having things happen *to* them. It's about creating a sense of safety and predictability, one gentle moment at a time.

Non-verbal communication is even more important with children. Sitting at eye level, using a calm voice, smiling gently, or engaging in a game or drawing session before treatment — these strategies help build rapport. Storytelling and play can also be powerful tools to help demystify procedures. I've often used hand puppets or character analogies to walk kids through what will happen during a visit, allowing them to feel more in control and less afraid.

Ultimately, children deserve to be treated with the same level of respect we give to adults. That means acknowledging their fears, listening when they say "no," and being honest in a way they can understand. Respect builds safety, and safety builds trust. And when children feel safe in the dental chair, we're not just making today's appointment easier — we're shaping a positive relationship with healthcare that can last a lifetime.

That said, not every clinician is naturally suited to working with children — and that's completely okay. Paediatric care requires patience, flexibility, and a certain lightness in approach. If you find yourself easily frustrated or unable to adapt to a child's pace and needs, it's far better — for both you and the patient — to refer to a colleague who thrives in that space. A negative early experience can have a lasting impact, so making sure the child is seen by someone who can support them with genuine care and understanding is always the right call.

Communicating well with kids is a skill, and like any other clinical skill, it can be learned and refined if desired. Training programs, workshops, or even simple role-play can go a long way in building the confidence to work with children. Whether it's learning how to explain procedures in age-appropriate language or managing fear-based behaviour with calm reassurance, this kind of preparation helps clinicians approach paediatric care with more empathy, patience, and emotional intelligence. And when we feel more confident, kids pick up on that too.

INCLUDING FAMILIES IN THE PROCESS

Whether supporting an older adult or a young child, families are often at the heart of care. They carry history, insight, and emotional weight. Including families in conversations, acknowledging their concerns, and inviting their input into care decisions fosters trust and strengthens outcomes.

In paediatric settings especially, parents or guardians are often navigating their own anxieties while trying to stay strong for their child. Taking the time to check in with them — to say, "How are you doing with all this?" — can mean the world. It reminds them that their emotional experience matters too.

I often speak to parents before their child's first dental visit to gently guide how they set expectations. While well-intentioned, parents can sometimes project their own past dental fears onto their children without even realising it. I encourage them to speak positively about the visit — say things like, "You'll get to go for a ride on the dental chair," or "The dentist will count your teeth, and you get to wear some really cool sunnies!" I suggest avoiding phrases like, "Don't be scared," or "It won't hurt," because children are incredibly perceptive and tend to pick up on the underlying anxiety in our tone and words. Setting the tone with curiosity and calm confidence can go a long way in shaping a child's view of healthcare for years to come.

The appointment doesn't end when the child hops off the chair. I often share take-home strategies or suggest fun resources — like brushing apps, interactive charts, or books about visiting the dentist — that can make oral care a positive part of a child's daily life. Giving parents tools they can use outside the clinic helps bridge the gap between appointments and empowers them to reinforce good habits in a fun, low-pressure way. It's all about supporting them for the whole journey, not just the visit in front of us.

Similarly, in aged care, adult children may be balancing the demands of caregiving with work, parenting, and guilt. Recognising these emotional undercurrents allows us to support the whole family unit, not just the patient. When we take a moment to ask, listen, and include, families feel valued — and when families feel supported, patients do too. Shared care planning is about creating a true sense of agency and partnership. When parents feel like collaborators, not just bystanders, they're more empowered to continue care confidently at home.

True partnership with families also means offering them a seat at the table. Involving them in care decisions — whether it's creating a shared care plan, asking for their insight into what comforts or unsettles their child, or simply taking time to explain what's coming next — strengthens trust and improves outcomes. When we treat parents as experts on their own child and support them with tools and resources to continue the experience positively at home, we reinforce their role as empowered advocates, not just passive observers.

CARING FOR OURSELVES IN EMOTIONALLY DEMANDING SETTINGS

These types of care — slow, intimate, emotionally complex — can take a quiet toll if we're not careful. Emotional labour isn't always loud, but it's always real. Being a consistent emotional presence for someone in decline or supporting a frightened child through procedures calls for immense compassion, but it also demands boundaries and self-awareness.

Regular debriefing with team members, access to mental health support, or simply stepping outside for fresh air and a moment of grounding can make all the difference. In long-term care settings, burnout can sneak in unnoticed, especially when the emotional load is carried silently. In paediatric care, repeated exposure to suffering or loss can be quietly overwhelming. Supporting each other — openly and without judgement — is vital.

We also need to celebrate the moments of joy. The child who gives a shy high five after a successful appointment. The elderly resident who lights up at hearing their favourite song. These are not small things. These are the moments that matter. The ones that sustain us.

EMOTIONAL INTELLIGENCE AS A CONSTANT COMPANION

At its core, this kind of work isn't just about procedures or policies — it's about people. When we bring emotional intelligence into vulnerable care settings, we don't just improve outcomes — we elevate the experience of care itself. Whether we're supporting a resident in the slow rhythm of aged care, guiding a child through a daunting procedure, or advocating for someone who can't communicate clearly, our presence, empathy, and insight shape how safe, seen, and supported they feel.

Chapter 7

Sustaining Emotional Intelligence in Daily Practice

Emotional intelligence isn't something we switch on for difficult moments and then leave behind. It's a daily discipline—woven into how we think, communicate, lead, and care for others. Throughout this book, we've explored how emotional intelligence strengthens our connections with patients, enhances collaboration within our teams, helps us navigate conflict and stress, and supports our own well-being and growth as clinicians.

In many ways, emotional intelligence is a lifelong practice. It's not about always getting it right, but about noticing, reflecting, recalibrating—and showing up with intention and authenticity. This final chapter offers a toolkit to help you carry these principles forward in the real-world chaos of healthcare. You don't need hours of spare time or a perfect system—just the willingness to pause, pay attention, and engage with yourself and others on a deeper level.

DAILY PERSONAL EI HABITS

The more we check in with ourselves, the better we show up for others. Emotional self-awareness is a habit, not a one-off event. As we saw in earlier chapters, even subtle shifts—like naming your emotional state or taking a moment to breathe—can create space between stimulus and response. This space is where regulation, empathy, and wisdom live.

Some clinicians start their day by asking, "How am I feeling right now, and how might that affect how I interact today?" Others close their day with a short reflection: What went well? What challenged me? What am I learning about myself?

These check-ins don't need to be formal. They might take the form of a few lines in a journal, a quiet moment over a cup of tea, a walk around the block between patients, or a breath-focused reset in the car before heading home. Mindfulness practices, gratitude statements, and emotional grounding rituals can all help regulate your nervous system and keep your EQ sharp. What matters is consistency, not perfection.

TEAM-BASED EI HABITS

Emotional intelligence thrives in teams where psychological safety, trust, and empathy are the norm. One emotionally aware individual can influence a culture—but real transformation happens when EI is embedded in the team's rhythm.

Start small. Begin team huddles or meetings with a one-word emotional check-in. This simple act encourages self-awareness and connection, helping each team member feel seen and supported.

Create space for feedback—not just performance-related, but emotional. "How did that conversation land for you?" or "Is there anything we could do differently next time?" These questions show vulnerability, invite collaboration, and model a culture of curiosity over criticism.

We've explored throughout the book how emotionally intelligent leadership isn't about titles or authority—it's about presence, trust-building, and emotional awareness. Whether you're in a formal leadership role or not, you can help model these practices and support your team to thrive emotionally, not just function operationally.

REFLECTION AND ASSESSMENT TOOLS

If you're looking to build on what you've learned, there are several tools that can deepen your self-awareness. Formal assessments like the Emotional Quotient Inventory (EQ-i 2.0) or the Emotional Competence Inventory (ECI) offer structured insights into your emotional strengths and areas for growth.

But you don't need a formal test to continue evolving. Informal reflection and honest peer feedback can be just as powerful. Try asking a trusted colleague:

- "What's one thing you see me do well when it comes to emotional awareness or empathy?"
- "What's one area you think I could work on?"

These kinds of conversations take courage, but they often reveal blind spots—and strengths—you may not realise you have.

Other helpful tools include:

- Emotional journaling prompts to track patterns and progress
- The Feeling Wheel to expand emotional vocabulary and clarity
- Weekly debriefs or peer reflections to unpack high-stress or emotionally complex cases in a psychologically safe space

Sustaining emotional intelligence isn't about mastering it once—it's about revisiting it often, with humility, honesty, and intention.

EMOTIONAL INTELLIGENCE ENHANCEMENT PLAN

To help bring all of this together, I've created a simple worksheet you can use to keep emotional intelligence front of mind. You'll find it on the Book Resources page at drlorabanicevic.com. It includes space for:

- Weekly self-check-ins
- Daily intention setting
- Reflective journaling prompts
- Feedback logs
- Small goals for incorporating EI into patient and team interactions

Print it out and keep it somewhere handy—on your desk, in your journal, or tucked into your bag. It's not about perfection; it's about giving yourself a small moment to stay grounded and intentional in how you show up each day.

A FINAL NOTE

As you move forward, remember: the work of emotional intelligence is never done—but that's part of its beauty. It grows with you. Whether you're managing a full ward, supporting a single patient, or navigating your own burnout and boundaries, these skills will help you lead, heal, and thrive.

Sustaining emotional intelligence isn't about being endlessly composed or perfectly empathetic. It's about committing to show up —open, reflective, and willing to grow—even when things are hard. These tools won't prevent every conflict or fix every challenge, but they will help you stay connected to the heart of your work. And in healthcare, where connection is everything, that makes all the difference.

You're not alone in this journey. Every emotionally intelligent moment, however small, creates ripples that benefit your patients, your colleagues, your loved ones, and yourself.

Keep showing up. Keep learning. Keep leading with heart.

Conclusion

Dear fellow clinician,

As we come to the end of this journey together, I want to take a moment to reflect — not just on the ideas we've explored, but on what it all means in practice.

Emotional intelligence in healthcare isn't just a nice bonus or an optional soft skill. It's foundational. It shapes the way we connect with patients, the way we communicate with our teams, and the way we care for ourselves. At its core, emotional intelligence helps us do what we came into this profession to do: help people feel safe, seen, and supported.

Throughout this book, we've unpacked what emotional intelligence really looks like in a clinical setting. We've looked at how self-awareness helps us manage our own emotional responses — those moments when stress rises or frustration creeps in — and how empathy allows us to better understand and connect with the people we serve. We've talked about how to build trust from that very first patient interaction, how to navigate difficult conversations with compassion, and how to lead teams with authenticity and care.

We've also explored some of the harder stuff — burnout, compassion fatigue, boundary-setting, and the emotional toll that can come with being "the strong one" day after day. These conversations matter. Because no matter how clinically skilled or technically brilliant we are, we can't pour from an empty cup. Emotional intelligence gives us tools not just to show up better for others — but to show up better for ourselves, too.

You've heard my stories — some light-hearted, some hard-won — and I hope they've reminded you that none of us have this completely figured out. I still get it wrong sometimes. I'm still learning. And that's the point. Emotional intelligence isn't a destination. It's a practice. A way of being. A lens we bring to every interaction, every challenge that comes our way, every appointment with a patient, every meeting with our team.

If there's one thing I hope you take away from this book, it's this: emotional intelligence isn't separate from clinical care. It *is* clinical care. It's the tone of your voice, the way you handle a setback, the pause before reacting, the choice to lean in when someone needs you most. And the ripple effect of that? Better outcomes for our patients, stronger relationships both inside and outside of work, a more sustainable, fulfilling career and personal well-being.

When I first opened my practice, my mission was to change the way people felt about going to the dentist. Along the way, I realised that what was missing — not just in dentistry but across the broader healthcare professions — was emotional intelligence. By bringing awareness to this and building these skills, we have the power to transform not only our patients' experiences, but our own as healthcare professionals.

So, what now?

Start small. Choose one skill to focus on. Reflect on your triggers. Try a new listening strategy. Debrief with your team. Be kind to yourself. And keep practicing. Because the kind of culture we all want to work in — the one that values empathy, presence, and psychological safety — starts with how each of us shows up every day.

Thank you for coming on this journey with me. I'm cheering you on as you bring these ideas into your own world — to your clinic, your team, your patients and beyond. The work you do matters. And how you do it? That matters even more.

If you'd like to connect, share your thoughts, or learn more about emotional intelligence in healthcare, you can find me at drlorabanicevic.com or follow me on social media @drlorabanicevic. I'd love to hear from you.

With heartfelt gratitude and unwavering belief in our collective potential,
Lora

Acknowledgments

I've always loved books. Last year alone, I read 72 of them — no small feat while raising a family, running a business, and juggling life's many moving parts. Books have been my teachers, my mirrors, and my companions. They've challenged my thinking, opened my heart and mind, and inspired me in more ways than I can count. Writing this one has been my way of giving back — to offer something of value, to pay it forward, and to hopefully inspire others the way so many authors have inspired me.

To my husband Jake — my rock, my safe place, and my greatest support — thank you. You married a strong and ambitious woman, and somehow, I seem to dream a little bigger every year. You never flinch at the chaos or the curveballs — instead, you meet them (and me) with steady calm and quiet strength. Your unwavering trust and belief in me — no matter how wild or untested my ideas may be — mean everything. You are a wonderful husband, an incredible father, and the truest partner I could ever ask for. I couldn't be the woman I am, or the one I strive to become, without you by my side — grounding me, cheering me on, and holding space for it all.

To my beautiful daughters, Liliana and Montana — everything I do is for you. You are the light of my life and the reason I strive to grow, create, and lead with heart every day. I want you to grow up knowing that you can achieve whatever you set your minds to if you are determined, focused, gritty, and unafraid to fail. Never giving up, especially when things get hard, is what truly sets you apart. Mistakes aren't something to fear — they are stepping stones to growth, resilience, and self-discovery.

I hope this book shows you that passion and purpose can live alongside kindness, compassion, and humility. That success isn't measured by titles or trophies — but by how we treat others and stay true to ourselves. These are lessons I learned from my own incredible grandparents, parents, and sister, who shaped me with their love, wisdom, and quiet strength. Thank you all for everything.

To my team at Corner 32 Dental — you are the heart of our practice. I'm so proud of the culture we've built together over the years: one rooted in kindness, support, fun, and positivity. We spend so much of our lives at work, and I feel genuinely blessed to have shared — and to continue sharing — those hours with such wonderful people. Whether past, present, or future team members, your passion, care, and good energy have helped shape this place and inspire me daily to be a better person and a better leader. You make me laugh every day, and I'm so grateful for all that you bring to our community.

To my best friends — Elena, Lorne and Olessia. Over two decades of friendship through every high and low...what a gift. You're like sisters to me, and once you've shared this much life with someone, you're bonded for life. Your love, humour, and unwavering support keep me grounded, and I'm so grateful to have you by my side — and to be by yours — as our lives continue to evolve.

To my coaches and now friends, Vicky Samios and Helen Skazas — your guidance and encouragement made this book possible. Thank you for believing in me, pushing me to keep going, and celebrating every small win along the way. And to my mentor, Aaron Sansoni — thank you for showing me what's possible when you dream bigger. To the entire Empire Circle community, thank you for the endless support, inspiration, and belief in what we're all building.

Finally, to you — the reader — and to every healthcare professional I've met along the way, and those I've yet to meet: thank you. Your dedication, heart, and daily efforts to care for others are what inspired this book in the first place. I hope it supports you, uplifts you, and reminds you of the power you hold — not just as a clinician, but as a human being.

With love and gratitude,
Lora

References

American Medical Association. (n.d.). What role does humor play in health care? Retrieved May 28, 2025, from https://www.ama-assn.org/delivering-care/ethics/what-role-does-humor-play-health-care

Beach, M. C., & Inui, T. (2006). Relationship-centered care: A constructive reframing. *Journal of General Internal Medicine, 21*(S1), S3–S8. https://pubmed.ncbi.nlm.nih.gov/16405707/

Berman, A. C., & Chutka, D. S. (2005). Assessing effective physician-patient communication skills: "Are you listening to me, doc?" *Mayo Clinic Proceedings, 80*(3), 338–343. https://pmc.ncbi.nlm.nih.gov/articles/PMC4951737/

Birks, Y. F., & Watt, I. S. (2007). Emotional intelligence and patient-centred care. *Journal of the Royal Society of Medicine, 100*(8), 368–374. https://pmc.ncbi.nlm.nih.gov/articles/PMC1939962/

Birkhäuer, J., Gaab, J., Kossowsky, J., Hasler, S., Krummenacher, P., Werner, C., & Gerger, H. (2017). Trust in the health care professional and health outcome: A meta-analysis. *PLOS ONE, 12*(2), e0170988. https://doi.org/10.1371/journal.pone.0170988

Borg, J. (2010). *Body language: 7 easy lessons to master the silent language* (pp. 94–95). Pearson Education.

Burgess, L. A., & Taylor, M. (2017). Increasing emotional intelligence through self-reflection journals. *Journal of Occupational Therapy Education, 1*(3), Article 6. https://encompass.eku.edu/cgi/viewcontent.cgi?article=1142&context=jote

Cairns, P., Pinker, I., Ward, A., Watson, E., & Laidlaw, A. (2021). Empathy maps in communication skills training. *The Clinical Teacher, 18*(2), 142–146. https://doi.org/10.1111/tct.13270

CareerStaff Unlimited. (2023, August). *Crisis management in healthcare: 4 strategies for facilities.* https://www.careerstaff.com/healthcare-staffing-blog/healthcare-staffing/crisis-management-in-healthcare-strategies/

Carnegie, D. (1936). *How to win friends and influence people.* Simon and Schuster.

Cifra, C. L., Sittig, D. F., & Singh, H. (2021). Bridging the feedback gap: A sociotechnical approach to informing clinicians of patients' subsequent clinical course and outcomes. *BMJ Quality & Safety, 30*(7), 591–597. https://doi.org/10.1136/bmjqs-2020-012464

Codier, E., & Codier, D. (2015). A model for the role of emotional intelligence in patient safety. *Asia-Pacific Journal of Oncology Nursing, 2*(2), 112–117. https://doi.org/10.4103/2347-5625.157594

Covey, S. R. (1989). *The 7 habits of highly effective people: Powerful lessons in personal change.* Free Press.

Crucial Learning. (n.d.). *Healthcare Resource Center.* Retrieved May 28, 2025, from https://cruciallearning.com/resource-center/healthcare

Derksen, F., Bensing, J., & Lagro-Janssen, A. (2013). Effectiveness of empathy in general practice: A systematic review. *British Journal of General Practice, 63*(606), e76–e84. https://doi.org/10.3399/bjgp13X660814

Gauthier, T., Meyer, R. M. L., Grefe, D., & Gold, J. I. (2015). Implementation of mindfulness training for mental health staff. *Mindfulness, 6*(4), 861–872. https://link.springer.com/article/10.1007/s12671-014-0330-2

Geisel School of Medicine at Dartmouth. https://geiselmed.dartmouth.edu/news/2023/more-than-words-body-language-and-patient-communication/

Gharaee, H., Jahanian, R., Hamidi, Y., Soltanian, A. R., Heidari Pahlavian, A., & Erfani, H. (2019). How much emotional intelligence effect on health centers performance? A structural equation modeling approach. *Journal of Research in Health Sciences, 19*(3), e00455. https://www.ncbi.nlm.nih.gov/pmc/articles/PMC7183552/

Guyon, L. (2023, December 12). *Improving professional learning through feedback loops*. Digital Promise. https://digitalpromise.org/2023/12/12/improving-professional-learning-through-feedback-loops/

Hall, L. H., Johnson, J., Watt, I., Tsipa, A., & O'Connor, D. B. (2016). Healthcare staff wellbeing, burnout, and patient safety: A systematic review. *PLOS ONE, 11*(7), e0159015. https://doi.org/10.1371/journal.pone.0159015.

Hardavella, G., Aamli-Gaagnat, A., Saad, N., Rousalova, I., & Sreter, K. B. (2017). How to give and receive feedback effectively. *Breathe, 13*(4), 327–333. https://doi.org/10.1183/20734735.009917

Henderson, C., Evans-Lacko, S., & Thornicroft, G. (2013). Mental illness stigma, help seeking, and public health programs. *American Journal of Public Health, 103*(5), 777–780. https://doi.org/10.2105/AJPH.2012.301056

Jahromi, V. K., Tabatabaee, S. S., Abdar, Z. E., & Rajabi, M. (2016). Active listening: The key of successful communication in hospital managers. *Electronic Physician,* 8(3), 2123–2128. https://doi.org/10.19082/2123

James, T. A. (2023, January 12). *Building empathy into the structure of health care.* Harvard Medical School. https://postgraduateeducation.hms.harvard.edu/trends-medicine/building-empathy-structure-health-care

Jasper, M. (2013). Reflective practice in health care and how to reflect effectively. *Nursing Times,* 109(24), 14–17. https://www.ncbi.nlm.nih.gov/pmc/articles/PMC5673148/

Jiménez-Picón, N., Romero-Martín, M., Ponce-Blandón, J. A., Ramírez-Baena, L., Palomo-Lara, J. C., & Gómez-Salgado, J. (2021). The relationship between mindfulness and emotional intelligence as a protective factor for healthcare professionals: Systematic review. *International Journal of Environmental Research and Public Health, 18*(10), 5491. https://doi.org/10.3390/ijerph18105491

Kashdan, T. B., Barrett, L. F., & McKnight, P. E. (2015). Unpacking emotion differentiation transforming unpleasant experience by perceiving distinctions in negativity. Current Directions in Psychological Science, 24(1), 10-16. https://psycnet.apa.org/record/2015-07847-002

Kashdan, T. B., Ferssizidis, P., Collins, R. L., & Muraven, M. (2010). Emotion differentiation as resilience against excessive alcohol use: An ecological momentary assess-

ment in underage social drinkers. Psychological Science, 21(9), 1341-134. https://pubmed.ncbi.nlm.nih.gov/20696854/
Kircanski, K., Lieberman, M. D., & Craske, M. G. (2012). Feelings into words: Contributions of language to exposure therapy. Psychological Science, 23(10), 1086-1091. https://pubmed.ncbi.nlm.nih.gov/22902568/
Knaak, S., Mantler, E., & Szeto, A. (2017). Mental illness-related stigma in healthcare: Barriers to access and care and evidence-based solutions. *Healthcare Management Forum,* 30(2), 111–116. https://doi.org/10.1177/0840470416679413
Kopynec, S. (2018, May 1). *Provider burnout and the risk of malpractice.* American Academy of Physician Associates. https://www.aapa.org/news-central/2018/05/provider-burnout-and-the-risk-of-malpractice/
Kriakous, S. A., Elliott, K. A., Lamers, C., & Owen, R. (2021). The effectiveness of mindfulness-based stress reduction on the psychological functioning of healthcare professionals: A systematic review. *Mindfulness,* 12(1), 1–28. https://doi.org/10.1007/s12671-020-01500-9
Lane, R. D. (2000). Levels of emotional awareness: Neurological, psychological and social perspectives. In R. Bar-On and J. D. A. Parker (Eds.), Handbook of emotional intelligence. Jossey-Bass. https://psycnet.apa.org/record/2001-00355-008
Lane, R.D., Sechrest, L., Riedel, R.G. Weldon, V. Kaszniak, A.W. & Schwartz, E.G. (1996). Impaired verbal and nonverbal emotion recognition in alexithymia. Psychosomatic Medicine, 58, 203-210. https://pubmed.ncbi.nlm.nih.gov/8771618/
Lewis, S., Willis, K., Bismark, M., & Smallwood, N. (2022). A time for self-care? Frontline health workers' strategies for managing mental health during the COVID-19 pandemic. *SSM Mental Health,* 2, 100053. https://doi.org/10.1016/j.ssmmh.2021.100053
Mabona, J. F., van Rooyen, D., & ten Ham-Baloyi, W. (2022). Best practice recommendations for healthy work environments for nurses: An integrative literature review. *Health SA Gesondheid,* 27, 1788. https://doi.org/10.4102/hsag.v27i0.1788
Matthews, G., Zeidner, M., & Roberts, R. D. (2002). Emotional intelligence: Science and myth. MIT Press.
McCreaddie, M., & Payne, S. (2012). Humour in health-care interactions: A risk worth taking. *Health Expectations,* 17(3), 332–344. https://doi.org/10.1111/j.1369-7625.2011.00758.x
McCreaddie, M., & Wiggins, S. (2008). The purpose and function of humour in health, health care and nursing: A narrative review. *Journal of Advanced Nursing,* 61(6), 584–595. https://doi.org/10.1111/j.1365-2648.2007.04548.x
Moudatsou, M., Stavropoulou, A., Philalithis, A., & Koukouli, S. (2020). The role of empathy in health and social care professionals. *Healthcare,* 8(1), 26. https://doi.org/10.3390/healthcare8010026
Murray, K. (2025, March 17). *Active listening: 10 tips to support someone with health issues.* British Heart Foundation. https://www.bhf.org.uk/informationsupport/heart-matters-magazine/wellbeing/how-to-talk-about-health-problems/active-listening

Nandyal, S., Strawhun, D., Stephen, H., Banks, A., & Skinner, D. (2021). Building trust in American hospital-community development projects: A scoping review. *Journal of Community Hospital Internal Medicine Perspectives, 11*(4), 439–445. https://doi.org/10.1080/20009666.2021.1929048

Ng, I. K., Tan, B. C., Goo, S., & Al-Najjar, Z. (2024). Mental health stigma in the medical profession: Where do we go from here? *Clinical Medicine*, 24(1), 100013. https://doi.org/10.1016/j.clinmc.2024.100013

Nightingale, S., Spiby, H., Sheen, K., & Slade, P. (2018). The impact of emotional intelligence in health care professionals on caring behaviour towards patients in clinical and long-term care settings: Findings from an integrative review. *International Journal of Nursing Studies,* 80, 106–117. https://doi.org/10.1016/j.ijnurstu.2018.01.006

Oliveros, E., Brailovsky, Y., & Shah, K. S. (2019). Communication skills: The art of hearing what is not said. *JACC: Case Reports, 1*(3), 446–449. https://doi.org/10.1016/j.jaccas.2019.09.003

Overton, A. R., & Lowry, A. C. (2013). Conflict management: Difficult conversations with difficult people. *Clinics in Colon and Rectal Surgery,* 26(4), 259–264. https://doi.org/10.1055/s-0033-1356728

Pond Jr, R. S., Kashdan, T. B., DeWall, C. N., Savostyanova, A., Lambert, N. M., & Fincham, F. D. (2012). Emotion differentiation moderates aggressive tendencies in angry people: A daily diary analysis. Emotion, 12(2), 326-337. https://pubmed.ncbi.nlm.nih.gov/22023359/

Prado, K., Robinson, A., & Chao, Y. Y. (2023). The impact of mindful meditation on health care workers during the COVID-19 pandemic. *Journal of Nurse Practitioners, 19*(3), 104513. https://doi.org/10.1016/j.nurpra.2022.11.023

Prezerakos, P. E. (2018). Nurse managers' emotional intelligence and effective leadership: A review of the current evidence. *The Open Nursing Journal, 12*, 86–92. https://doi.org/10.2174/1874434601812010086

Raecke, J., & Proyer, R. T. (2022). Humor as a multifaceted resource in healthcare: An initial qualitative analysis of perceived functions and conditions of medical assistants' use of humor in their everyday work and education. *International Journal of Applied Positive Psychology,* 7(3), 397–418. https://doi.org/10.1007/s41042-022-00074-2

Robinson, L., Segal, J., & Smith, M. (n.d.). *Emotional Intelligence Toolkit.* HelpGuide.org. https://www.helpguide.org/articles/mental-health/emotional-intelligence-toolkit.htm

Ryan, R. M., & Deci, E. L. (2001). To be happy or to be self-fulfilled: A review of research on hedonic and eudaimonic well-being. In S. T. Fiske (Ed.), *Annual review of psychology* (Vol. 52, pp. 141–166). Annual Reviews. https://pubmed.ncbi.nlm.nih.gov/11148302/

Salovey, P., & Mayer, J. D. (1990). Emotional intelligence. Imagination, cognition and personality, 9(3), 185-211. https://journals.sagepub.com/doi/10.2190/dugg-p24e-52wk-6cdg

Schutte, N. S., Malouff, J. M., Thorsteinsson, E. B., Bhullar, N., & Rooke, S. E. (2007). A meta-analytic investigation of the relationship between emotional intelligence and health. Personality and Individual Differences, 42(6), 921-933. https://www.sciencedirect.com/science/article/abs/pii/S0191886906003539

Shamay-Tsoory, S. G., Harari, H., Aharon-Peretz, J., & Levkovitz, Y. (2013). Emotional intelligence and prefrontal cortex: A comparative study of the Wisconsin Card Sorting Test (WCST) performance in patients with frontal lobe lesions and normal subjects. *Iranian Journal of Psychiatry,* 8(1), 12–19. https://www.ncbi.nlm.nih.gov/pmc/articles/PMC3939963/

Sheikhrabori, A., Peyrovi, H., & Khankeh, H. (2022). The main features of resilience in healthcare providers: A scoping review. *Medical Journal of the Islamic Republic of Iran,* 36, Article 3. https://pmc.ncbi.nlm.nih.gov/articles/PMC9386779/

Shouhed, D., Fang, A., & Daskivich, T. J. (2019). Association of emotional intelligence with malpractice claims. *JAMA Surgery,* 154(3), 250–251. https://pubmed.ncbi.nlm.nih.gov/30698614/

Šimić, G., Tkalčić, M., Vukić, V., Mulc, D., Španić, E., Šagud, M., Olucha-Bordonau, F. E., Vukšić, M., & Hof, P. R. (2021). Understanding emotions: Origins and roles of the amygdala. *Biomolecules,* 11(6), 823. https://doi.org/10.3390/biom11060823

Simões de Almeida, R., Costa, A., Teixeira, I., Trigueiro, M. J., Rocha Dores, A., & Marques, A. (2023). Healthcare professionals' resilience during the COVID-19 and organizational factors that improve individual resilience: A mixed-method study. *Health Services Insights,* 16, 11786329231198991. https://doi.org/10.1177/11786329231198991

Squires, A. (2018). Strategies for overcoming language barriers in healthcare. *Nursing Management,* 49(4), 20–27. https://doi.org/10.1097/01.NUMA.0000531166.24481.15

Sutton, J. (2023, September 7). *Mirror neurons and the neuroscience of empathy.* PositivePsychology.com. https://positivepsychology.com/mirror-neurons/

Symplr. (n.d.). *How healthcare leaders can improve workforce morale.* https://www.symplr.com/blog/how-healthcare-leaders-can-improve-workforce-morale

USF Health. (n.d.). *Goal-setting strategies for healthcare professionals.* USF Health Online. https://www.usfhealthonline.com/resources/career/goal-setting-strategies-for-healthcare-professionals/

Weng, H.-C. (2008). Does the physician's emotional intelligence matter? Impacts of the physician's emotional intelligence on the trust, patient-physician relationship, and satisfaction. *Health Care Management Review,* 33(4), 280–288. https://doi.org/10.1097/01.HCM.0000318765.52148.b3

Willcox, G. (1982). The feeling wheel: A tool for expanding awareness of emotions and increasing spontaneity and intimacy. Transactional Analysis Journal, 12(4), 274-276. https://doi.org/10.1177/036215378201200411

Zeidner, M., Matthews, G., & Roberts, R. (2009). What we know about emotional intelligence: How it affects learning, work, relationships and our mental health. MIT Press. https://doi.org/10.7551/mitpress/7404.001.0001

Made in the USA
Monee, IL
26 June 2026

55825701R10173